WITHDRAWN

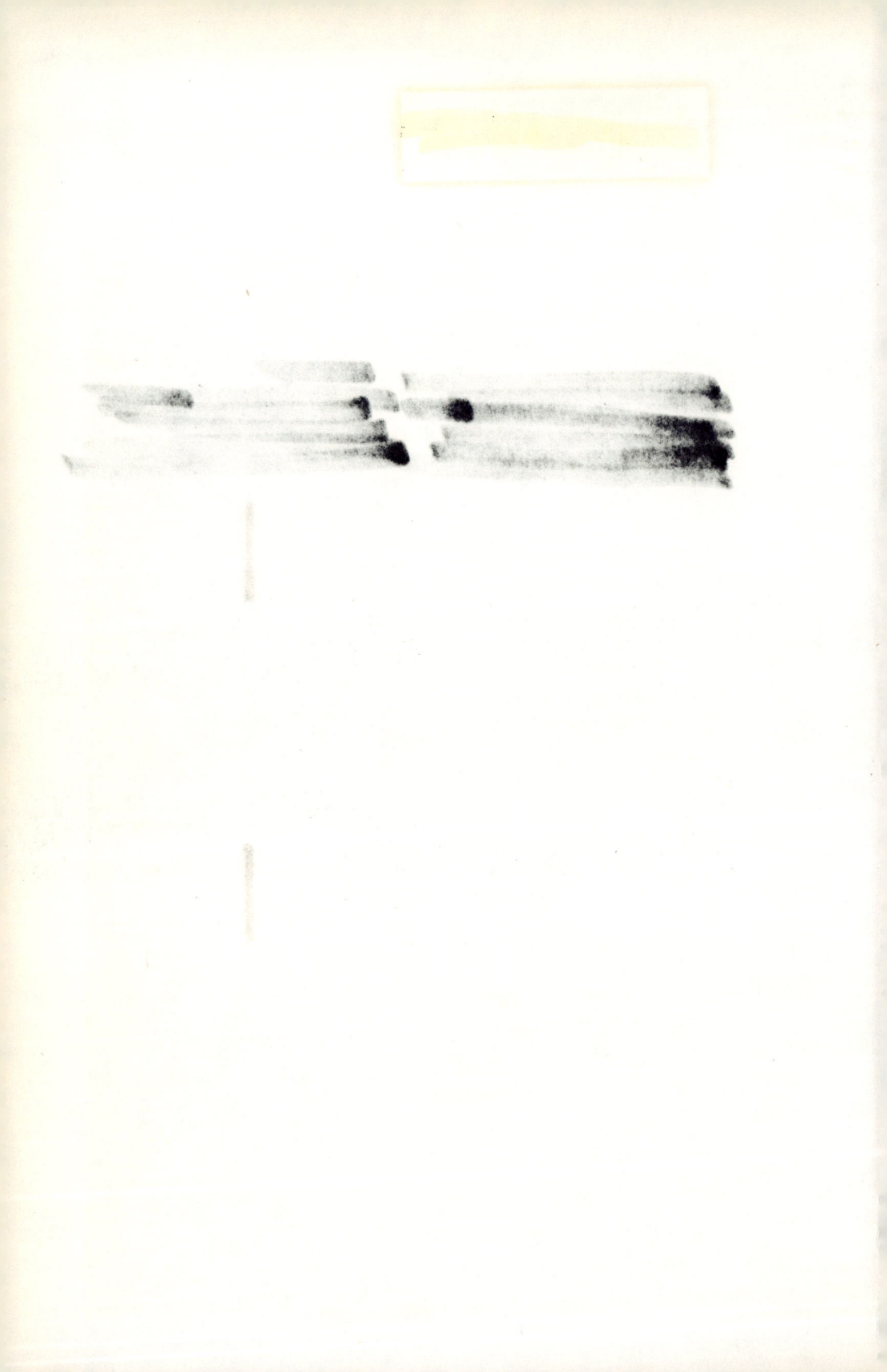

Extending Life, Enhancing Life

A National Research Agenda on Aging

Committee on a National Research
Agenda on Aging

Edmund T. Lonergan, Editor

Division of Health Promotion and
Disease Prevention

INSTITUTE OF MEDICINE

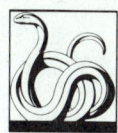

NATIONAL ACADEMY PRESS
Washington, D.C. 1991

NATIONAL ACADEMY PRESS • 2101 Constitution Avenue, N.W. • Washington, D.C. 20418

NOTICE: The project that is the subject of this report was approved by the Governing Board of the National Research Council, whose members are drawn from the councils of the National Academy of Sciences, the National Academy of Engineering, and the Institute of Medicine. The members of the committee responsible for the report were chosen for their special competencies and with regard for appropriate balance.

This report has been reviewed by a group other than the authors according to procedures approved by a Report Review Committee appointed by the members of the National Academy of Sciences, the National Academy of Engineering, and the Institute of Medicine.

The Institute of Medicine was chartered in 1970 by the National Academy of Sciences to enlist distinguished members of the appropriate professions in the examination of policy matters pertaining to the health of the public. In this, the Institute acts under both the Academy's 1863 congressional charter responsibility to be an adviser to the federal government and its own initiative in identifying issues of medical care, research, and education.

Support for this study was provided by the Commonwealth Fund (Grant No. 9221) and the Pew Charitable Trusts (Grant No. 86-06646-000). In all cases, the statements made and the views expressed are those of the National Academy of Sciences, Institute of Medicine, and do not reflect those of the Commonwealth Fund or the Pew Charitable Trusts.

Library of Congress Cataloging-in-Publication-Data

Institute of Medicine (U.S.). Committee on a National Research Agenda on Aging.
    Extending life, enhancing life : a national research agenda on aging / Committee on a National Research Agenda on Aging, Division of Health Promotion and Disease Prevention, Institute of Medicine : Edmund T. Lonergan, editor.
        p.   cm.
    Includes bibliographical references and index.
    ISBN 0-309-04399-9
  1. Aging—Research. 2. Aging—Research—Government policy—United States. I. Lonergan, Edmund T. II. Title.
    QP86.I56 1991
    362.1'9897'0072073-dc20   91-2947
                                                                                             CIP

This book is printed on acid-free recycled paper.

Copyright: © 1991 by the National Academy of Sciences

Printed in the United States of America

    The serpent has been a symbol of long life, healing, and knowledge among almost all cultures and religions since the beginning of recorded history. The image adopted as a logotype by the Institute of Medicine is based on a relief carving from ancient Greece, now held by the Staatlichemuseen in Berlin.

*DeWITT S. GOODMAN, Director, Institute of Human Nutrition, and Professor of Medicine, Columbia University College of Physicians and Surgeons, New York, New York

*WILLIAM N. KELLEY, Executive Vice President and Dean, University of Pennsylvania Medical Center, Philadelphia

GEOFFREY PLACE, Vice President, Research and Development, Procter and Gamble Company, Cincinnati, Ohio

THOMAS D. POLLARD, Professor of Cell Biology and Anatomy, Johns Hopkins University School of Medicine, Baltimore, Maryland

JOHN E. ROBSON, Deputy Secretary, Department of the Treasury, Washington, D.C.

*JOHN W. ROWE, President, Mount Sinai School of Medicine, and President, Mount Sinai Hospital, New York, New York

*JUDITH RODIN, Philip R. Allen Professor of Psychology; Chair, Department of Psychology; and Professor of Medicine and Psychiatry, Yale University, New Haven, Connecticut

ROBERT J. RUBIN, President, Health and Sciences Incorporated, Washington, D.C.

*FRANK A. SLOAN, Centennial Professor of Economics and Chairman, Department of Economics, Vanderbilt University, Nashville, Tennessee

Chief Consultant to the Committee and Coordinator, Liaison Teams

LESTER SMITH, Associate Professor of Medicine, Department of Medicine, Section on Geriatrics/Gerontology, Howard University College of Medicine, Washington, D.C.

Institute of Medicine

GARY B. ELLIS, Director, Division of Health Promotion and Disease Prevention
**EDMUND T. LONERGAN, Study Director
JOSEPH S. CASSELLS, Senior Staff Officer

---

*IOM member.
**Affiliation: Associate Chief of Staff for Geriatrics and Chief, Geriatric Section, Department of Veterans Affairs Medical Center; Clinical Professor of Medicine, University of California, San Francisco.

Committee on a National Research Agenda on Aging

*JULIUS R. KREVANS (*Chair*), Chancellor, University of California, San Francisco
*JOHN E. AFFELDT, Medical Advisor, Beverly Enterprises, Rancho Santa Fe, California
PATRICIA ARCHBOLD, Professor and Chair, Department of Family Nursing, Oregon Health Sciences University, Portland
*BEN D. BARKER, Professor and Dean, School of Dentistry, University of North Carolina, Chapel Hill
STANLEY J. BRODY, Emeritus Professor of Physical Medicine and Rehabilitation in Psychiatry, University of Pennsylvania Medical Center, Philadelphia
ANTHONY CERAMI, Professor and Head, Laboratory of Medical Biochemistry, Rockefeller University, New York, New York
VINCENT J. CRISTOFALO, Audrey Meyer Mars Professor and Director, Center for Gerontological Research, The Medical College of Pennsylvania, Philadelphia
*CARROLL L. ESTES, Professor and Chair, Department of Social and Behavioral Sciences, Director, Institute of Health and Aging, University of California, San Francisco
CALEB FINCH, Arco/William S. Kieschnick Professor in the Neurobiology of Aging, University of Southern California, Los Angeles

LINDA A. DePUGH, Administrative Assistant
***RICHARD WILLIAMS, Program Assistant
THEODORA FINE, Contract Editor

Advisers to the Committee

ROBERT N. BUTLER, Brookdale Professor and Chairman, Department of Geriatrics and Adult Development, Mount Sinai Medical Center, New York, New York
DOROTHY P. RICE, Professor in Residence, University of California School of Nursing, San Francisco
ALEXANDER RICH, Sedgwick Professor of Biophysics, Massachusetts Institute of Technology, Cambridge
T. FRANKLIN WILLIAMS, Director, National Institute on Aging, National Institutes of Health, Bethesda, Maryland
ROSALYN S. YALOW, Solomon Berson Distinguished Professor at Large, Mount Sinai Medical Center, and Senior Medical Investigator, Department of Veterans Affairs Medical Center, Bronx, New York

Consultants

SUSAN COZZENS, Department of Scientific and Technological Studies, Rensselaer Polytechnic Institute, Troy, New York
JACOB J. FELDMAN, Associate Director for Analysis and Epidemiology, National Center for Health Statistics, Hyattsville, Maryland
GAIL JACOBY, Chief, Office of Planning, Technological Information, and Research, National Institute on Aging, Bethesda, Maryland
KATHRYN HYER, Associate Director, Health Care Policy Unit, Ritter Department of Geriatrics, Mount Sinai Medical Center, New York, New York
TIM MEYER, Market Analyst in Pharmaceutical Research and Development, Procter and Gamble Company, Cincinnati, Ohio
GARY MIRANDA, Technical Writer/Editor, Kaiser Permanente Health Research, Portland, Oregon
SUSAN PHILLIPS, Research Associate, San Francisco, California

---

***Affiliation: Department of Veterans Affairs Medical Center, San Francisco, California.

Preface

In 1988, with generous support from The Commonwealth Fund and The Pew Charitable Trusts, the Institute of Medicine (IOM) convened a committee of 18 national authorities on health care to develop priorities on age-related research for the next 20 years, and to estimate the resources required to carry out the new research agenda. The IOM also asked the committee to identify research that would enhance the understanding of basic processes of aging and maximize function in older persons; to alert scientists to promising but neglected areas of research on aging; and to bring the importance of age-related research to the attention of government, academic institutions, industry, and the public.

Impetus for this study was provided by two major themes: (1) the opportunity furnished by the potential of science to improve the quality of life and independence of our older citizens and (2) the need to respond to the growing numbers of dependent and demented persons 65 years of age and over.

The committee was aided by 63 outstanding scientists comprising 4 liaison teams—basic biomedical research, clinical research, behavioral and social research, and health services delivery research—and by 2 experts in biomedical ethics (see Appendix A). Further guidance was provided by 5 senior advisors to the committee and by input from more than 60 leaders in the field of health care and aging. Liaison teams and the experts on biomedical ethics prepared documents for the committee's use, and the committee met 4 times over a 2-year period to create the current report.

The present work can be seen as an extension of earlier studies by the National Institute on Aging: *Our Future Selves*, in 1978,[1] and *Toward an Independent Old Age: A National Plan for Research on Aging*, in 1982.[2] These reports described the promise of science to meet the burdens posed by a growing population of disabled older persons and presented an *extensive* list of research opportunities in the study of aging.

The current study offers a *limited* number of general research priorities for the coming decades. To carry out this program the committee recommends a significant increase in the funding of approved research grants on aging, expansion of training of faculty in age-related studies, widening of the scientific infrastructure base, and additions to present centers for the study of aging.

More than 150 health care professionals contributed to this report. The committee wishes to express its gratitude to Samuel O. Thier, president of the IOM, for his steadfast support of this complex project. The study initially went forward with support from Enriqueta C. Bond, the IOM executive officer, and was continued and brought to conclusion with the assistance of Gary B. Ellis, director of the IOM's Division of Health Promotion and Disease Prevention.

This report is restricted to the committee's description of the opportunities and advantages of increased research on aging. Given that resources are available, the committee would suggest that expenditures on research related to aging be increased as recommended in the report. The report does not, however, consider the effects of a large increase in spending on aging research on other U.S. health and human welfare-related research, and the committee realizes that resources are not unlimited. In addition, the committee does not comment on the desirability of increasing expenditures on research on aging versus expenditures on research on children, cancer, AIDS, contraception, the brain, or other major areas of investigation involving health care of younger adults. This report should not be used to determine priorities in the *general* area of health research, nor is it intended to set priorities for *all* health-related research.

---

[1] National Institute on Aging, *Our Future Selves* (Bethesda, Md.: U.S. Government Printing Office, 1978).

[2] National Institute on Aging, *Toward an Independent Old Age: A National Plan for Research on Aging* (Bethesda, Md.: U.S. Government Printing Office, 1982).

In closing, it should be noted that the dictionary defines "agenda" as "a list of things to be done," and it is in this sense of the word that the current work is presented. The program outlined in the following pages states the committee's commitment to the concept that increased fundamental research on aging holds the most promise to improve the lives of an ever-increasing number of older Americans. It is now the task of the leaders of this country—in government, foundations, industry, education, and science—to join with an informed public to evaluate and implement this program.

>Julius R. Krevans, Chairman
>Committee on a National Research
>Agenda on Aging

Contents

Executive Summary and Recommendations for Funding 1
   Background, 4
   A National Research Agenda on Aging, 9
   Crosscutting Issues, 24
   Recommendations for Funding the Research Agenda on Aging, 26
   Implications for Funding Agencies, 35
   Concluding Comments, 37

1 Introduction 40

2 Basic Biomedical Research 47
   Research Priorities, 49
   Additional Research Opportunities, 50
   Resource Recommendations, 52
   Crosscutting Issues, 55

3 Clinical Research 57
   Research Priorities, 58
   Additional Research Opportunities, 66
   Resource Recommendations, 67
   Crosscutting Issues, 68

4 Behavioral and Social Sciences 71
   Justification and Major Themes, 72
   Research Priorities, 75
   Additional Research Opportunities, 80
   Methodological Needs, 81
   Resource Recommendations, 82
   Cross-Disciplinary and Crosscutting Issues, 83

5 Health Services Delivery Research 88
   Long-Term Care and Continuity of Care for Older Persons, 90
   Financing of Health Care for Older Persons, 95
   Drug Use, 96
   Mental Health Services, 99
   Disability/Disese Prevention and Health Promotion Services, 100
   Research Priorities, 101
   Additional Research Opportunities, 102
   Resources Required, 102
   Cross-Disciplinary and Crosscutting Issues, 103

6 Research in Biomedical Ethics 107
   Research Priorities, 107
   Additional Research Opportunities, 115
   Conclusions and Resource Recommendations, 115

7 Review of Resources Committed to Research on Aging 119
   Funding Support for Research on Aging, 119
   Institutions Engaged in Research on Aging, 123
   Publications on Research in Aging, 125
   Personnel Engaged in the Study of Aging, 127

Appendixes

A Acknowledgments 135
   Liaison Teams, 135
   Experts Providing Information to the Committee, 140
   Directors, DVA Geriatric Research, Education, and
   Clinical Centers, 142
   Directors, Pharmaceutical Company Research, 143

B Background Documents 144

Index 145

Executive Summary and Recommendations for Funding

Science offers the best hope to improve the older person's quality of life. Research that is directed and supported properly can provide the means to reduce disability and dependence in old age, and can decrease the burdens on a health care system strained to its limits.

This is a time for celebration but a time as well for deep concern. It is a time for celebration because gains in life expectancy have resulted in an estimated 33 million Americans 65 years old and over, the majority of whom are vigorous and active well into advanced old age. It is a time for concern because, for a growing number of older people and their families, these added years of life often are burdened by disability, dementia, and the loss of independence.

In testimony before the Committee on a National Research Agenda on Aging, Joseph A. Califano, former Secretary of Health, Education, and Welfare, said:

> The aging of America will challenge all our political, retirement, and social service systems. As never before, it will test our commitment to decent human values. Nowhere is the aging of America freighted with more risk and opportunity than in the area of health care.

The urgent need to respond to this risk is underscored by census figures showing that the subgroup of older persons most vulnerable to disability and dementia, those 85 years of age and over, is growing six times faster than the rest of the population, and by evidence indicating that the cost of caring for disabled older persons will more than double in the coming decades unless the causes of disability can be identified and controlled (Schneider and Guralnick, 1990).

The following themes of risk and opportunity have guided the preparation of this report, and have justified support for the study of aging through scholarship and research:

1. the need to control acute and chronic illness in old age and to achieve a major reduction in disability and suffering, thus not merely extending life but enhancing it; and

2. the new opportunity offered by science to improve the quality of life for older persons through analysis and discovery of the relationships among basic biological phenomena, disease, economic and social deprivation, disability, and dependence.

Building on two reports by the National Institute on Aging (NIA), *Our Future Selves* (1978), and *Toward an Independent Old Age: A National Plan for Research on Aging* (1982), the present agenda aims to identify priority research on aging in basic biomedical science, clinical science, and behavioral and social studies as they relate to health, health services delivery, and biomedical ethics. To this end, the Institute of Medicine (IOM) convened a committee of 18 leaders in national health care, and charged them to:

- identify for the next two decades priorities in research on aging that will contribute to the quality of life and maximize the independence of older persons;
- stimulate research on the fundamental processes of aging and the prevention of disability and disease, and further the application of current knowledge to the treatment of age-related disorders;
- alert scientists to promising but neglected areas of research on aging;
- provide the stimulus that will encourage new investigators to undertake the study of aging, and continue to engage the interest of established researchers in this field;
- estimate the resources required to fulfill the scientific needs for gerontological and geriatric research;
- guide federal and nonfederal funding agencies in supporting this research, and identify collaborative and nonduplicative funding patterns for government, industry, and private sources of support; and
- bring the importance of research on aging to the attention of government, private institutions, industry, the scientific community, and the public at large.

During the project the committee became convinced of the importance of ethical issues in clinical care and research on aging, and added this topic to the agenda.

Four liaison teams aided the committee: **basic biomedical research, clinical research, social and behavioral research,** and **health services delivery research**. Each of the teams was comprised of experts in their respective fields. Recommendations on **biomedical ethics** were provided by two national authorities in this field.

The reports of the liaison teams (see Appendix B) served as a major resource for the committee's deliberations. Guidance also was provided by five senior advisors who have made major contributions to the field of health care. Lastly, advice from experts in private foundations, government, industry, national organizations, and scientific institutions was obtained. The report, although assisted by information provided by more than 150 authorities, is the product of the committee's critical analysis of information received and represents the independent decisions of the committee.

Committee members and liaison team leaders developed criteria to identify priority research topics. Although different fields of study emphasized different criteria, in general, priority research areas were selected for their potential to:

- contribute to the understanding of the basic mechanisms of aging;
- address problems of disability and functional impairment in older persons;
- increase knowledge both of the interaction between disease and aging and of age-related diseases;
- lower morbidity and mortality rates among older persons;
- be implemented in a timely and feasible manner, with short-term goals achievable in 5 years or less and long-term goals achievable in 5 to 20 years;
- lead to cost reduction in health care;
- increase knowledge of behavioral and social factors in health and disease, and help older people maintain social as well as biological health;
- improve pharmacologic treatments of patients; and
- attend to relatively neglected areas of investigation.

The 1982 *Toward an Independent Old Age: A National Plan for Research on Aging* lists more than 350 research possibilities; the present committee's agenda is restricted to 15 areas of priority research. As conceived, the research priorities listed in this report represent the conceptual issues that underlie the questions and specific propositions of research proposals. The committee notes that in developing research priorities all five of the research areas were felt to be of first-rank importance, and the committee emphasizes that support should extend across all five of the fields of age-related research described in this report. Within each field of research, priorities are ranked according to their importance to the understanding of aging and their potential to improve the quality of life for older persons.

A national research agenda on aging has a broad multidisciplinary view, but it must be selective. The charge by the IOM dictated an agenda with the most promise for substantial impact on the individual during the next two decades—that is, research on the health and functioning of older individuals.

BACKGROUND

Support for Training and Research in Geriatrics and Gerontology

At the heart of health care for the older population are the educational programs that train the professionals who can respond to the health problems of elderly persons and make the scientific discoveries that will improve the quality of life of the later years. A 1980 study predicted that by the year 1990 training would be needed to produce 7,000 to 10,300 geriatricians to provide care for older persons having the most complex geriatric problems—those 75 years of age and over (Kane et al., 1980).

Programs for training have not met this goal, as shown by the finding that by the mid-1990s there will be only 5,000 certified geriatricians in this country (Reuben et al., 1990). To train an adequate number of geriatricians, Kane et al. (1980) estimated a full-time geriatric faculty of 1,230 to supervise hospital training programs in internal medicine or family practice, plus 370 to staff medical schools, and 450 for geropsychiatry, totaling about 2,100 faculty members and comprising both academic clinicians and researchers.

A 1987 IOM study, commenting on the small number of geriatric training programs (under 5 percent of all postgraduate medical programs), found that these programs graduated about 100 fellows per year and recommended that to meet needs for biomedical faculty by the year 2000 the number of graduates per year should be raised to at least 200 (IOM, 1987). Another study found training programs far short of goals for the year 2000 to develop nonbiomedical (mainly behavioral and social scientists) faculty in aging (National Institute on Aging, 1987). The serious shortage of faculty and researchers in age-related fields requires prompt attention by organizations that have traditionally supported this training (National Institute on Aging; Department of Veterans Affairs; National Institute of Mental Health).

Although training programs on aging, initially supported by the National Institute of Mental Health and the National Institute of Child Health and Human Development, began in the 1950s and 1960s, the establishment of the National Institute on Aging, the development of research and training programs in aging by the Department of Veterans Affairs, and the growth of scores of university programs in this country have taken place for the most part since 1970. Many discoveries in aging arising from this national effort—from molecular biology to behavioral and social science—await application to health problems and to improvement of function in older people.

Support is needed to continue these advances. The 1990 budget of the National Institutes of Health (NIH) devoted about $442 million, or about 6 percent of all funds, to the study of aging, with about $239 million coming from the NIA (including funds for research grants, centers, education, and demonstration projects) and an additional $203 million for research on aging coming from other parts of the NIH (Office of Planning, Technology, Information, and Evaluation, NIA). In 1990 other federal departments and agencies (see Chapter 7 for details) provided additional funds of about $144 million for research on aging. Foundations added $15 million in support. The National Pharmaceutical Association lists $3.6 billion for research and development on drugs used to treat diseases occurring in older patients, but it is difficult to know how much of this money was designated for age-related research as such.

An increase in funding for research on aging could produce rapid advances in the ability to respond to the problems of many older persons. For example, the neurosciences are poised to make major discoveries in Alzheimer's disease, but for every 100 dollars spent on care for the victims of this disease, under 0.5 percent, or less than 50 cents, goes to research that might lead to the control of Alzheimer's disease (Advisory Panel on Alzheimer's Disease, 1989).

A recent article underscored the effect of restricted funds on research, noting that at the NIA the funding rate of approved traditional investigator-initiated research projects (R01s) for fiscal year 1989 was 16.9 percent, or about one in six (Movsesian, 1990). This percentage and that of all funded approved research project grants on aging (24 percent) are slightly lowered due to reapplications (see the latter discussion in the section on recommendations for funding).

Low funding rates for research grants diminish opportunities for developing careers in age-related studies and may contribute to undersubscription to training programs in geriatrics (IOM, 1987).

In 1990 support for research on aging from all sources (NIH + Department of Veterans Affairs + other federal departments and agencies + foundations), described further in Chapter 7, amounted to an estimated $601 million, or less than 0.5 percent of the estimated 1987 (the most recent year for which figures are available) $162 billion cost of care for disability and illness in older patients (Waldo et al., 1989). This small national commitment to research in aging is a wasteful strategy in light of the potential contribution of research to improve the status of older persons and to reduce the enormous and expanding costs of their care.

A growing sense of urgency is accompanied by the recognition that the time is right to bridge the gap between the needs of an aging society and the scientific knowledge base. The nation now needs a comprehensive plan for research on aging. By identifying research priorities and the resources to support research on aging, it is the committee's intent to respond to that need.

The Aging Society:
Current Costs for Health Care of Older Persons

Most older persons are vigorous and have lives of good quality, and more than 50 percent of those 80 years and over are independent in self-care. Although mortality rates have fallen in the older generation, with increasing life expectancy, chronic diseases have become a major cause of death and disability. For instance, Rice reported that 40 percent of persons 75 and over had two or more chronic illnesses and that the proportion of the aged population reporting multiple chronic conditions had risen in recent years (Rice, 1989).

Of the 10 leading causes of death among older persons, only 2— heart disease and diabetes mellitus—are listed among the 10 leading chronic geriatric conditions (National Center for Health Statistics, 1989). Most of the leading chronic conditions involve disability and prolonged decline. Disability here is defined as any restriction on or impairment in performing an activity in the manner or within the range considered normal for a human being (World Health Organization, 1982).

Chronic conditions contributing to disability include arthritis, heart disease, strokes, disorders of vision and hearing, nutritional deficiencies, and oral-dental problems (in up to 40 percent of older persons; Baum, 1988). Dementia (especially Alzheimer's disease), not listed as a leading cause of death or disability in older persons, nevertheless for those 75 years and older is a major contributor to disability, nursing home placement, and, indirectly, to mortality rates (Weiler, 1987).

Fewer than 7 percent of persons aged 65 to 74 require assistance with dressing or bathing. At 75 to 84, these activities require help in 7 percent to 14 percent of older persons, and at 85 and beyond, up to 30 percent will need help with bathing (National Center for Health Statistics, 1987). Nursing home placement is needed for those who lack social supports and are most limited in ability to care for themselves. One half of nursing home residents require assistance with five or more activities of daily living (ADLs: bathing, dressing, grooming, transferring from bed to chair, going to the bathroom, being continent, feeding oneself), but for every one of the 1.4 million in skilled nursing facilities, two equally impaired older adults are receiving care at home.

The cost of health care for older persons is great and growing rapidly. In 1987 the cost to provide health care for elderly patients was $162 billion or $5,360 per capita, compared with $45.2 billion ($1,856 per capita) a decade earlier (Waldo et al., 1989). Medicare costs alone were almost $75 billion for the care of disability and illness among old people in 1987, and they may rise to $145 billion per year (in 1987 dollars) by the year 2020 (Schneider and Guralnick, 1990).

Sick older people are burdened by accelerating costs for their own care. In 1980 the average yearly expenditure by older persons for health care was $966, and in 1988 it was $2,394. Costs for medical care borne by older people have more than doubled in the past decade and may triple in the coming decade (Select Committee on Aging, 1990).

The Potential of Research on Aging

The description of the compression of morbidity in old age (Fries, 1980), with the older person collapsing suddenly after many years of vigor, has stimulated a closer study of the relationship between morbidity and mortality in old age. In 1986 a 65-year-old person could look forward to 17 more years of life and an 85-year-old to 6 more years. By contrast, *active* life expectancy, which implies ability to care for oneself and be independent, was only 10 years for 65 to 70-year-olds, and for 85-year-olds it was only 2.9 years (Katz et al., 1983).

Diminishing mortality rates thus may swell the ranks of sick and debilitated elderly persons, and the number of years of dependent old age may increase, with ever greater outlays for health and medical care (Gruenberg, 1977; Schneider and Guralnick, 1990). Like Tithonus, to whom the god Zeus gave eternal life without eternal youth (Graves, 1955), long life is a punishment if the quality of the later years is poor.

A model developed by Manton describes the potential of intervention to improve the quality of life for older persons. If medical care fails to diminish the incidence of disease among older persons, therapy that reduces lethal complications of disease may increase life expectancy in this group, but at the high cost of prolonging chronic illness and associated disability. Therefore, basic research should aim to promote interventions that decrease mortality by diminishing the incidence, severity, and rate of progression of disease. This approach will then improve *active* life expectancy as well as life expectancy, with slowing of the rate of "aging," and with increased independence among older individuals (Manton and Soldo, 1985; Soldo and Manton, 1988; Fries, 1990). An example of this kind of intervention is seen in the recent advances in the prevention and treatment of the chronic degenerative disorder osteoporosis, and related hip fractures in older women.

The power of research to reduce health costs dramatically usually is underestimated. The lifetime cost to maintain two Rh brain-damaged children or two children severely crippled by poliomyelitis (and there were thousands of these children in 1960) was greater than all of the money spent on the research that virtually eliminated these conditions (J. Krevans, University of California, San Francisco, personal communication, 1990). Postponing by one month the onset of severe disability that leads to nursing home placement for older persons could lead to savings of $3 billion per year, minus the cost of providing care for these patients at home. This is based on 1987 figures (the most recent available) for nursing home costs of $32.8 billion per year for those 65 years of age and over (Waldo et al., 1989), adjusted for inflation to $36 billion for 1990.

The committee is convinced that basic research, properly supported and directed, holds the promise to decrease chronic illness and disability in old age, enriching the quality of life and maintaining vigor and independence in the later years.

A NATIONAL RESEARCH AGENDA ON AGING

Basic Biomedical Research

While the term *aging* can apply to changes occurring during any phase of life, *dysfunctional aging* (or *senescence*) refers to changes associated with accelerated morbidity and mortality rates during the latter phase of adult life. Biomedical studies on the disorders of senescence include not only specific disease states but also conditions not easily classified. Basic biomedical science can substantially improve the quality of life for older persons, and add to the list of social and medical advances in which the nation takes pride, advances that eliminated so many of the killing and crippling diseases of childhood and younger adults.

A number of puzzling questions about aging have attracted the interest of biomedical researchers. Why do humans differ so individually in aging changes of bone, brain, and heart? What preconditions for aging may be set earlier in life, perhaps even in utero? What is the role of gene-environmental interactions in the individual patterns of aging? The committee believes that understanding these processes will lead to interventions that may delay or even reverse disability.

Although many fundamental processes of aging are yet to be understood, progress already has been made in distinguishing between the process of natural aging and disease states associated with older age. Achieving further knowledge will require contributions from genetics, biochemistry, cell biology, neurobiology, and other disciplines. Equally important is the integration of aging research with other areas of investigation that historically have focused on specific organs and diseases without considering the surrounding manifold of aging changes. The committee emphasizes that many major advances in science have been unanticipated. Therefore, it is essential to maintain the traditional primacy of investigator-initiated studies—the source of many research breakthroughs.

Recent advances in the basic biomedical study of aging will contribute significantly to the foundation for future progress in the understanding of how individuals age. Among these achievements are insights into gene regulation and other basic cellular functions; the development of colonies of rats that have shown increased lifespan and delayed decline of function following food restriction; and the creation of strains of mice with targeted mutations (i.e., basic changes in the genetic blueprint for proteins) that will improve understanding of the processes of aging.

Major conceptual and methodological successes in molecular biology will lead to high-resolution gene mapping and to increased understanding of gene expression at the molecular level. These advances have the potential for identifying the location and cloning of genes responsible for various age-related disorders, including familial Alzheimer's disease. It will then be possible to study how such genes may be controlled to prevent or further delay the adverse effects of age-related disorders.

The elucidation of the biological mechanisms of aging and the clinical and lifestyle interventions derived from these discoveries will improve the quality of advanced age. Moreover, such research findings are eminently achievable.

Priority Research Recommendations

For the 1990s and the first decade of the twenty-first century, planning and implementation of a multiinstitutional basic biomedical research effort in two principal areas should be undertaken.

Abnormal cell proliferation Research in this area involves the study of proliferative homeostasis, a fundamental process responsible for the orderly replacement of cells lost because of either exposure to toxins or endogenous processes (Martin, 1979). Mechanisms underlying pervasive disturbances in proliferative homeostasis that accompany aging in humans and other mammals are pivotal in many diseases that cause senescence. Alterations in cell replacement are vital to regeneration and repair, but they contribute to the genesis of many forms of cancer, atherosclerosis, osteoarthritis, benign prostatic hyperplasia, and disturbed immune function. The committee proposes that this major new national initiative be comparable in emphasis to the number one priority of the NIA—Alzheimer's disease and the neurobiology of aging.

Brain aging Basic research in the neurosciences (including the peripheral and central nervous systems) and the current special research initiatives on Alzheimer's disease should be continued and expanded.

Additional Research Opportunities

The research priorities in basic biomedical science listed above merit primary consideration for implementation, but other promising areas of biogerontological investigation, discussed at length in

Chapter 2, also merit support. Some of these important research directions are as follows:

- the study of the repair and regeneration of postmitotic nondividing cells, including neurons and cardiac and skeletal muscle cells, as well as conditionally proliferating cells, such as hepatocytes;
- the study of the major integrative systems of physiology, including the effects of aging on the immune and endocrine-neuroendocrine systems, the effect of dietary restriction on lifespan, and the regulation of reproductive and developmental physiology;
- the study of the varying rates of aging among different cells, tissues, and organs for individual differences within species and for species differences that will provide information about genetic influences;
- the study of the biomarkers of aging, their relationship to overall functional state, and the role of functional capacity as a marker of senescence;
- the study of the general question of gene expression in aging (especially as applied to the abnormal proteins associated with Alzheimer's disease or the inactivation of enzymes with age), selective changes in gene activity, and the effects of environmental influences on aging (e.g., free radicals, radiation, and various toxins); and
- the use of comparative genetics and development of new model systems to study aging and the lifespan.

The committee emphasizes that additional resources to support research on aging should supplement, not supplant, existing support for current basic research, either in aging or in other areas of biological investigation.

Resource Recommendations

First in importance, increase the funding of NIA—and other NIH—approved investigator-originated research proposals on aging from the present level of one in four to one in two.

- Increase the availability of animal models (including primates and other long-lived animals that more closely resemble humans) and laboratory animal models with contrasting maximal lifespans.
- Improve access to cell lines and tissue samples, especially cryopreserved cells and tissues, and cell and tissue types from different human populations that crosscut age, sex, and stages of disease (e.g., different stages of diabetes mellitus or Alzheimer's disease).
- Expand existing human longitudinal studies, making available

archival information from previous studies, including data on mortality rates and incidence of disease/disability from different human and animal populations.

- Add at least 10 Centers of Excellence in Geriatrics and Gerontologic Research and Training (Claude Pepper Centers) to the current three supported by the NIA (see funding section), in which multidisciplinary age-related studies can be carried out and in which high-technology tasks fundamental to a wide variety of research on aging can be supported.
- Increase support to train an additional 200 basic biomedical scientists per year in gerontology.

Clinical Research

The rapid growth of clinical research in geriatric medicine in the past decade has yielded new understanding of the physiology of aging, the mechanisms underlying many age-related disorders, the effectiveness of intervention to prevent or treat these disorders, and the characterization of frail elderly people, including those in long-term care. The committee has reviewed this database to identify two major priority areas to serve as the basis for specific research questions and proposals.

These priority areas, described below, overlap in some instances with interests shared by basic biomedicine and other fields of research, including the interest of behavioral/social studies and health services delivery in the study of the effectiveness of intervention in improving the health and function of older persons. This overlap illustrates the interdisciplinary character of age-related research.

Priority Research Recommendations

Research into the causes, prevention, management, and rehabilitation of functional disability in older persons, including a focus on the geriatric syndromes Functional disability in older persons is the major obstacle to independence, and 23 percent of older persons are impaired (less for those under 75; about 50 percent for those 85 and over) in one or more of the self-care activities that make independent existence possible (National Center for Health Statistics, 1985). The clinical research community currently is well positioned to make significant short-term advances leading to improvement in dependency and frailty in persons of advanced old age. This group is increasing rapidly in size and needs help urgently, especially in health promotion and disease prevention, and in studies of specific geriatric syndromes.

Health promotion and disease prevention in old age Although many research areas have been identified, two are offered as examples that show special promise for discovery. First, research should be conducted on the interacting effects of age, lifestyle, and disease on disability among older persons. Intervention studies should determine the changing effect of such factors in the prevention and rehabilitation of disability. Second, studies should examine the effectiveness of various disease prevention strategies for elderly persons and the extent to which preventive interventions may forestall late-life disabling conditions that begin in earlier life. Obviously, this research is interdisciplinary, overlapping with social and behavioral issues.

Studies of geriatric syndromes Although many syndromes are age associated, the five listed below offer unusually promising opportunities to benefit from careful clinical exploration. These syndromes are among the most prevalent of all late-life maladies.

- Failure to thrive: This syndrome involves poor nutrition, including decreased appetite and weight loss (often with dehydration), inactivity, depression, impaired immunity, and low cholesterol. One promising line of research is the conduct of crosscohort and longitudinal studies to determine true prevalence, risk factors, and precipitating events of this syndrome. Another important area is the study of interventions to prevent or treat poor nutrition and other factors associated with failure to thrive, such as pressure sores, increased infection, and depression.
- Impaired postural stability, muscle strength, and mobility: This widespread problem includes falls, dizziness, syncope (fainting), fractures, muscle weakness, and lack of mobility. Each year over one million older persons sustain fractures, including 200,000 hip fractures, that are related to this syndrome (Cummings et al., 1985). Recommended research includes (1) the study of pathophysiologic mechanisms and other factors (e.g., poor nutrition, auditory and visual impairments, and specific neurological defects) underlying recurrent falls and (2) the study of interventions, including drugs, that improve or further impair some of these functions.
- Mismanagement of medications: Polypharmacy, defined as the taking of three or more medications regularly, occurs in one-third of those over 65. Research in this area should include (1) studies of the fundamental pharmacodynamics of medications in older individuals

and (2) studies of medication use and effects that link discoveries in basic biomedicine (e.g., gene delivery systems, specific enzyme-blocking agents, and monoclonal antibodies) to clinical studies, behavioral investigation, and health services research.

• Urinary incontinence: Although the degree of urinary incontinence varies widely among individuals, this condition is present in approximately 30 percent of community-dwelling older persons (Diokno et al., 1986); 50 percent of those in nursing homes are incontinent (Ouslander et al., 1982). Urinary incontinence has major consequences in suffering and in costs of care among the older population. Behavioral, neuroanatomic, and neurophysiologic studies are needed to determine the basis of urinary incontinence and the efficacy and risk of currently available treatment modalities.

• Delirium: About one-third of hospitalized elderly individuals develop acute confusion, markedly complicating their hospital course and dramatically increasing morbidity and health care costs (Lipowski, 1989). Very little is known about the predisposing factors, natural history, underlying mechanisms, and effective treatment of delirium.

Studies of the interaction of age-dependent physiologic changes and important diseases in old age Research on the interaction between disease and aging is interdisciplinary, drawing on insights provided by research in molecular biology, physiology, nutrition, and behavioral and social science. This research may prove critical for issues of functional capacity, because the major diseases discussed below impose heavy burdens in old age and because better understanding of the linkage between age-related disease and disability may lead to improved independence in older people.

• Cardiovascular disorders: Cardiovascular disease is the major cause of death in older persons and is a leading cause of chronic illness and disability. Research should explore genetic and other risk factors as well as the molecular basis of atherosclerosis; the development of standard and recombinant-based drug technologies along with gene therapy approaches and nutritional interventions to treat or prevent hypertension and atherosclerosis; and evaluation over time of therapy for cardiovascular disease to assess cost benefits and effect on quality of life.

• Dementia and affective disorders: Dementia after age 75 affects 40 percent of the population (Hagnell et al., 1983) and is the major reason for disability among the very old. Great is the need for studies linking basic and clinical approaches to an understanding of the pathophysiology, cause, prevention, and treatment of Alzheimer's disease and other forms of dementia. These studies should include assessment of cellular and molecular markers as well as new approaches to imaging and neurotransmitter mapping of the nervous system. Affective disorders are underreported in old age, although they account for substantial disability (Finlayson and Martin, 1982). Multidisciplinary studies to investigate the pharmacology, neuroendocrinology, and behavioral and social aspects of affective disorders are recommended.

• Musculoskeletal disorders: Musculoskeletal disorders are second only to cardiovascular disease both as a cause of disability and as a cause of high health care costs among older persons. The application of techniques of powerful reverse genetics such as recombinant fragment length polymorphism (through which genes that contribute to serious genetic disorders such as cystic fibrosis have been found) will help to define the genetic basis of osteoarthritis and osteoporosis in many patients with these common disorders. This approach should receive a high priority as gene replacement techniques are developed as potential cures of such disorders. Other recommended research includes study of nutritional factors and nutritional therapy, and the investigation of the effectiveness of traditional and new rehabilitative interventions on musculoskeletal disorders.

• Infectious diseases and immunosenescence: Although infection is felt to play an important role in disability in older patients, further study is needed on the contribution of infection to disability and on the effect of prevention and treatment of infection in the older population. Further examples of research include topics such as whether vaccines can bypass the need for immune T cells and whether vaccines made with live attenuated organisms, vaccines with antiidiotypic antibodies, or vaccines with antigens attached to a rigid molecular backbone are effective in elderly persons. Efforts should utilize such new technologies as genetically engineered vaccines and attenuated viruses in studies in this important area.

• Neoplasia (cancer): Death from cancer is increasing among older persons; indeed, cancer is the second leading cause of lost years of life in the geriatric population. Although accumulation of mutations with age plays a major role in the emergence of neoplasia, more knowledge is needed to explain why age is the most important predictor of cancer in this group; nor is there sufficient information about the value of prevention and treatment of cancer in older patients. Reverse genetics (as described above), recombinant DNA products, and delivery systems using gene transfer approaches (mechanisms for inserting DNA into the body) should be especially valuable in this area. Finally, research into nutritional and other risk factors in the development of cancer should be expanded.

- Disorders of metabolism and homeostasis: Disorders of metabolism and homeostasis may precede and almost always influence the emergence and severity of the conditions described previously. The committee recommends studies on the pathophysiology and molecular genetics of conditions such as diabetes mellitus, altered muscle metabolism, altered bone and mineral metabolism, and altered lipid metabolism in old age.

Additional Research Opportunities

These include:

- investigation of the molecular biology, pathophysiology, prevention, and treatment of common sensory deficiencies of old age, especially impairment of hearing and vision;
- examination of the factors associated with oral and dental problems of old age, including periodontal disease, disorders of salivation, and oral-facial pain;
- study of common skin conditions of elderly persons, such as dry skin, itching, and predisposition to cancers of the skin; and
- study of the interaction between nutrition and normal aging and between nutrition and age-associated diseases.

Resource Recommendations

The support required for an effective research program in the priority research areas involves added funds, phased in over 5 years, most importantly an increase in the funding rate of NIH-approved investigator-initiated research grants on aging from one in four to one in two; provision of education and support for an additional 200 to 300 fellows and postdoctoral students and 100 to 150 junior faculty per year, coupled with necessary continued support for midlevel investigators new to the fields of geriatrics and gerontology; expansion of current infrastructure supports; and the addition of at least 10 new Claude Pepper Centers, as described more fully in the section on funding.

Behavioral and Social Research

Fundamental advances in the study of aging have shown that psychological and behavioral variables, along with factors in the social and physical environment, can alter the course of aging dramatically. Thus, the process of aging is highly responsive to social and behavioral interventions. Studies employing such interventions as training in cognitive skills or increasing the sense of competence and self-efficiency in some older individuals who are deficient in these qualities have had dramatic effects on function and health.

Research in the social and behavioral sciences has emphasized that aging is an interactive and lifelong process. This view also has provoked interest in the associations among biological differences, behavior and psychosocial processes, and alterations in physiological systems in health and disease.

The potential of the aging process to respond to modification provides a unique opportunity for future research. Individuals arrive at the end of life by quite different socially determined, as well as biologically determined, routes. Differentiation in older adults provides some of the best evidence for the modifiability of aging processes and the experience of aging. *Differentiation* refers to variability in aging, both within and across societies. Studies have found that behavioral capacities are multidirectional over the adult life course: some remain stable, and others decline or improve. Because individuals adjust to biological decline in aging, behavioral decline often is minimal.

Aspects of differentiation in elderly persons also involve variations in individual and cohort lifestyles, risks of illness and dependency, and functional capacity. Cultural and psychological processes influence the aging process in varied and consequential ways. Most studies documenting this influence have focused on reducing age-related decrements in health. Research is needed to specify the broader areas and limits of the modifiability of aging, emphasizing the enhancement of existing skills and the potential for learning new skills in later life.

Another major perspective in social and behavioral research focuses on the interaction between person and environment. Specific sociocultural contexts influence the aging process differently in specific individuals. Study of these contexts should include how aging differs across societies and across cultural, racial, and ethnic groups; how aging is influenced by differences in work place, treatment environment, living arrangements, and other material and social supports; and how individual capacity and social milieu affect behavior and health outcome.

Priority Research Recommendations

Three research priorities emerge from these themes.

Investigation of the basic social and psychological processes of aging, including specific mechanisms underlying the interrelation-

ships among social, psychological, and behavioral variables and between these variables and biological aging functions, should be undertaken Examples include investigation of the relationship between memory function and central nervous system structures such as between the hippocampus and cerebellum (Berger et al., 1986), and research on stress-related environmental, psychological, and hormonal factors that lead to anatomic changes in the brain (see cerebral atrophy following extreme stress: Jensen et al., 1982; Finch, 1987). Special attention should be paid to at-risk populations, such as women, the poor, and minorities, since study of these populations may lead to new understanding of the dynamic interaction between biological and social variables.

The relationship between brain and behavior represents an exciting new research frontier. Basic research is needed to provide a clearer understanding of individual differences in sensory, cognitive, and behavioral aging, particularly as these differences reflect relationships between brain and behavior, environment and behavior, and society and behavior. Clinical research should apply what is known about the modifiability of risk factors, skills, learning, and memory. Despite recognition that the major health problems of older people are chronic, little attention has been paid to behavioral and social interventions to reduce disability and provide new strategies for management. Research should address rehabilitative strategies, evaluate the social and emotional barriers to rehabilitation, and explore issues related to compliance.

Research that addresses issues of change in population, dynamics, and particularly the question of postponed morbidity is a further high priority Descriptive demography, epidemiology, and population estimates are especially important to forecast the number of older people who will be independent or not. New measures are needed to evaluate the sequence of disease and/or disabling impairment and death for individuals and social groups—compared by cohort over time. Research on the postponement of disability and dependence through changes in social context, and through behavioral intervention, must accompany studies of psychosocial predictors of health, longevity, and functional disability in the aged.

Psychological and behavioral variables may not only contribute to biological aging, but may also serve to mirror physiological dysfunction. In developed societies most older people are vigorous and independent, but certain groups of older adults (e.g., women and minorities) are at higher risk for poverty, social isolation, underemployment, inadequate education, illness, and inaccessibility to health care. Factors that postpone morbidity may function differently in these groups, making them especially important to study.

Research should be undertaken to study the manner in which societal structures and societal changes affect aging Just as individuals change, so too do social structures. Societal old age today shows neither what old age was like in the past nor what it will be like in the future. It is crucial to determine how stability and change in social structures such as the family and work place affect the performance, productivity, health, and quality of life of older adults. Retirement from work or major changes in family structure or in family roles such as the increased entry of women into the workforce provide an opportunity to study how social change affects the experience of aging and health and the well-being of older persons. Research should examine the implication of these changes for social support and caregiving.

Research is needed as well to specify what changes in social structure could improve productivity in older people. Changes in mandatory retirement laws urgently call for more understanding of productivity and psychological processes in older workers. Finally, a life-course perspective should be adopted that views younger adults as the older adults of the future. If children and younger adults who are underemployed, undereducated, and underinsured can be identified and helped, this may improve the well-being of the older population of the future.

Studies derived from the priority research areas identified above may involve large-scale, longitudinal investigations. At the same time, consideration should be given to exploring the use of small-sample studies to enhance our knowledge on key aspects of the aging process.

Additional Research Opportunities

Opportunities for social research include the following:

- study of the characteristics of employment, work places, and older individuals associated with continued productive activity in lifelong jobs or in new careers;
- study of how older people are affected (expected and actual performance) by changing technology, and how firms use training and job respecification to make technological changes as age neutral as possible; and
- development of a quality of life index to identify contributing

factors among subpopulations for whom the index is low (e.g., the very old and minorities).

Opportunities for behavioral research include the following:

- study of the psychological concomitants of illness and how these affect self-care and response to formal care;
- study of the comparative effectiveness of different modalities in the treatment of chronic mental disorders; and
- examination of the effect of behavioral and social intervention on the outcome of long-term illness.

Resource Recommendations

Despite increases in the federal commitment to health research, the social and behavioral sciences have lost ground relative to other areas of investigation. Support for behavioral and social research on aging in 1989 was estimated at $80–$100 million from the federal government and $10–$15 million from nonfederal sources such as foundations (Behavioral and Social Research Program, NIA). Estimates of resources for the research agenda primarily involve investigator-originated studies and are to be phased in over a 5-year period.

Behavioral and social research will require substantial added funds during the first 5 years of the new research agenda, especially to raise funding for approved NIH research proposals on aging from one in four to one in two. Because much of the support for behavioral and social studies in aging comes from agencies outside the NIH (e.g., the Health Care Financing Administration and the Alcohol, Drug Abuse, and Mental Health Administration), support for research on aging by non-NIH agencies should be increased by at least 50 percent.

Other support includes training for 200 more behavioral and social scientists per year, one-time costs for construction of additional centers for multidisciplinary research (see the recommendations for funding section), and a share in funds for infrastructure utilized by all areas of research on aging.

Health Services Delivery Research

The growth of the older population, particularly those 85 and over, the chaotic state of today's health care system, rising health care costs, and mounting public concern about value received for the health care dollar lend urgency to the need for a new impetus in health services delivery research. Research in health services delivery expands knowledge about the organization, financing, and deliv-

infrastructure funding. Because significant funding for health services delivery studies comes from outside NIH, additional funds are requested from agencies traditionally supporting this research (e.g., the Health Care Financing Administration and the Agency for Health Care Policy and Research).

Research in Biomedical Ethics

Ethical issues accompany all aspects of health care of older persons and are at the heart of research on this group. Areas of major importance in ethics and in the study of aging include the following: dilemmas regarding life-sustaining treatment, selection of therapeutic interventions based on age, distribution of health care resources, and the need to include older subjects in research. Prolonging life in some patients may not (or may) be desired by them or be appropriate; guidelines to establish responsibility for these decisions often are problematic for elderly persons. Competing social needs, growing costs of care, and the enlarging population of sick and disabled older persons pose problems of resource allocation that require agreement on how to make such determinations fairly. Finally, there is a need to determine the most ethical way to do research on older persons who are institutionalized, frail, or cognitively impaired.

Priority Research Recommendations

Funds should be provided to conduct analytical and empirical research on biomedical ethical issues in three priority areas:

Dilemmas regarding life-sustaining treatment
Allocations of health care resources
Participation in clinical research by frail elderly persons

Additional Research Opportunities

These opportunities include:

- study of clinician-patient interaction regarding life-sustaining technologies;
- research into decision making for incompetent patients who lack advance directives;
- study of the role of institutional ethics committees;
- the identification of medical futility;
- study of resolution of disagreements between caregivers and patients or their families;

- defining appropriate care standards for elderly persons;
- investigation of the use of age as a criterion for allocation of health services;
- study of ethics in day-to-day interaction between caregivers and older patients (e.g., autonomy of older patients); and
- research into the trade-off between quality of care and quality of life for older patients.

Resource Recommendations

Although the NIH National Center for Human Genome Research recently set aside 3 percent of its funds for the study of ethical issues, which could include ethical issues in the care of older persons, the committee knows of no other federal support for research on ethics and geriatric patients, and it strongly encourages funding in this area, following the model of the genome project in association with specific biomedical, clinical, social and behavioral, and health services delivery research projects.

CROSSCUTTING ISSUES

Crosscutting issues bridge the disciplines and call for an interdisciplinary approach to their study. Such issues include gender, ethnic origin, cultural background, ethics, race, and the interdisciplinary approach to training and scientific investigation.

Basic Biomedical Research

Major crosscutting issues here involve the study of the effect of race, gender, ethnic background, and other factors on the trajectory of aging, ranging from the cellular level to the intact organism. This study involves coordinated efforts with other disciplines to provide an integrated approach to multifactorial phenomena. The overarching issue of ethics applies to basic biomedical investigation in raising questions about the care and disposition of experimental animals and the application of new discoveries, such as gene transplants. Finally, interdisciplinary education in the area of gerontology/geriatrics should be supported.

Clinical Research

Clinical research on aging engages many disciplines. Insights from molecular and cell biology provide a basic biomedical foundation for much clinical research. Behavioral and social research along with health care delivery studies can facilitate clinical investigation of the response of older people to illness and of the effect of interventions to reduce disability and morbidity occurring late in life.

Of equal importance are crosscutting issues that involve gender, racial, and ethnic differences in response to illness, including how older persons experience illness, or in the metabolic disposition of drugs. It would be interesting to understand, for example, the marked difference in morbidity of blacks compared to whites with equal degrees of hypertension or of women compared to men insofar as hypertension-related morbidity is concerned. Another issue involves ethics in clinical research—a subject discussed in the previous section of this summary.

Behavioral and Social Research

Many crosscutting issues arise in behavioral and social research, including the effects of gender, race, and ethnicity on longevity, functional status, and morbidity in old age; social role expectations and appropriateness of intervention; and population dynamics to predict longevity and morbidity. In addition, neurobiological study of cognitive defects will be enriched by combination with approaches to intellectual function and its modifiability through behavioral and social intervention. Study in these areas requires interdisciplinary research that cuts across all of the areas of study described in this report, from basic biomedical to health services delivery.

Health Services Delivery Research

Significant differences in the utilization of health services by men and women extend beyond the distribution of chronic illnesses and morbidity in these groups. Gender differences are seen in participation in programs of prevention and in economic/social status of older persons. These variances should be investigated further. Other topics include the assessment of need for health services based on different patterns of illness and disability between men and women, gender influence on response to different modes of health care delivery, and sex differences in utility of common preventive and risk reduction interventions.

RECOMMENDATIONS FOR FUNDING THE RESEARCH AGENDA ON AGING

The committee believes that a major investment in research on aging is needed urgently and therefore recommends additional funds of about $312 million per year, not adjusted for inflation, phased in over a 5-year period. These funds, added to current research supports of approximately $601 million, total $913 million annually, a figure approaching the $1 billion recommended by the Pepper Commission (1990). In addition, a nonrecurring expenditure on construction of about $110 million will be required. Programs of research on aging and support for centers should continue to be funded on the basis of merit and the accepted high standards of competition for research funds.

To estimate added funds for the study of aging the committee used available data (e.g., costs for centers, research projects, and training); where substantiating evidence was limited, the committee's decisions were based on judgment.

The federal government bears most of the cost of health care for older persons and is the only institution with the resources and organization to provide the wide-ranging research support requested in this report. Foundations and industry will add to support for research on aging, but it is mainly to the federal government, especially for its support of NIH and other federal department and agency sponsored research on aging, that the committee's recommendations are directed.

It should be noted that in estimating funds for age-related research the committee did not consider the effects of a large increase in spending on research on aging on other U.S. health and human welfare-related research, and the committee realizes that resources are not unlimited. In addition, the committee does not comment on the desirability of increasing expenditures on research on aging versus expenditures on research on children, cancer, AIDS, contraception, the brain, or other major areas of investigation involving health care of younger adults. Although this report is not intended to set priorities in the general area of health research, or to set priorities for all health research, the recommendations for additional funding in this section follow from the committee's conviction that increased fundamental research on aging holds the most promise to improve the lives of the ever-increasing numbers of older Americans.

Table 1 summarizes the National Research Agenda on Aging. The additional resources required to develop this agenda include research project grants, centers for the study of aging, funds for infrastructure, construction for centers and infrastructure, and training of new

TABLE 1 National Research Agenda on Aging: Summary of Research Priorities

Research Area	Research Priorities
Basic biomedical research	Abnormal cell proliferation The aging brain
Clinical research	Functional impairment and disability Interaction of age-dependent physiological changes and disease
Behavioral and social research	Interaction of social, psychological, and biological factors in aging Changes in population dynamics; the postponement of morbidity Changes in societal structures and aging
Health services delivery research	Long-term care and continuity of care Costs and financing of long-term care Medications and older persons Mental health services Disability and disease prevention and health promotion
Biomedical ethics	Dilemmas involving life-sustaining treatment Allocation of health care resources Participation of older persons in research

SOURCE: Institute of Medicine, 1991.

investigators. Funds required to obtain these resources are summarized in Table 2. Additional funds to support the research agenda have not been adjusted for inflation and are to be phased in over a 5-year period.

Derivation of Recommendations for Funding

Funds for Research Projects

Major achievements in the health sciences are rarely predictable, but have usually come from the laboratories of gifted investigators exploring basic research questions. These advances often require the support of research originating from individual researchers or from small groups of investigators. Therefore, the preeminent expansion

TABLE 2 Summary of Additional Funds (rounded off in millions of dollars) Needed for the Research Agenda

Resource Support	Funds Needed
Increased NIH funding of research project grants	$ 92
Funding for cooperative clinical trials	25
Non-NIH research support for behavioral/social and health services delivery research	80
Increased support for training of scientists	50
Infrastructure	50
Centers of Excellence	15
Total	$312
Construction	$110

NOTE: Funds are for yearly funding of resources, except for construction funds. Construction funds are a one-time cost. All estimates are in current dollars.

of support for the research agenda on aging must be a major increase in funding for approved age-related research project grants (RPGs), especially the traditional investigator-initiated proposals (R01s) by the NIA and other branches of the NIH.

In fiscal year 1990 the average funding of approved RPGs at the NIH was 25 percent (4,917/18,956); at the NIA funding of approved RPGs was 24 percent (192/799) (Office of Information Systems Branch, Division of Research Grants, National Institutes of Health). The percentage of funding for approved RPGs is slightly lowered by the presence of reapplications. For example, in fiscal year 1990 at the NIA 30 percent of the approved RPG applications (241/799) were resubmissions. The NIA funding rate for approved reapplications was 23 percent (55/241), and for first-time applications was 25 percent (137/558); the lower rate of funding of reapplications slightly diminished the overall funding rate of approved RPGs to 24 percent. A similar small effect of reapplications on the percentage of funding of approved RPGs was seen for the total number of RPGs funded by the NIH.

To improve support for this most important source of discoveries in aging, the committee recommends that funding of approved RPGs in aging by the NIA and other divisions of the NIH should be increased from the current level of one in four to one in two. In addition, although the U.S. House of Representatives has recently advised that the average NIH funding cycle be limited to 4 years, because of the long duration of chronic illness and disability characteristic of aging, the committee urges that more review cycles for research on aging be extended to 5 to 7 years.

To increase the funding of approved RPGs on aging, the committee recommends an additional $92 million per year for this purpose, to be phased in over 5 years. The committee suggests that a significant part of this increase should be made available as soon as possible in order to take advantage of high-quality projects ready for implementation and also to provide early encouragement to scientists interested in entering the field of studies on aging. The increase in funding applies to RPGs at the NIA and to RPGs on aging approved by other branches of the NIH.

In fiscal year 1990 NIA support for 192 RPGs (at $190,000 per RPG) was $36.5 million, or about 17 percent of the total NIA budget of $239 million (Budget Office, NIA). The percentage of funds devoted to RPGs at the NIA was higher than the overall 12 percent ($945 million/$7.6 billion) of the total NIH budget funding of all RPGs for fiscal year 1990 (Division of Research Grants; Reports, Analysis, and Presentation Section, NIH).

The committee was unable to obtain information about the number of non-NIA-funded RPGs on aging, but estimated a minimum number of about 294 RPGs. This estimate was based on an average cost of $190,000 per RPG per year and assignment to age-related RPGs of 30 percent, or $55.8 million, of the $186 million committed to research on aging by non-NIA institutes in fiscal year 1990 (see Table 7-1). This is a conservative estimate: the actual funding and number of these non-NIA RPGs may have been higher because the non-NIA institutes committed fewer dollars to training and other non-research project supports of studies on aging than did the NIA. Given the estimate of non-NIA support for RPGs on aging, the figure of about $92 million in additional funds can derived from the following calculations:

Funding of approved RPGs on aging: funding level—one in four

- NIA $36.5 million (192 RPGs)
- NIH $55.8 million (294 RPGs)
- Total $92.3 million (486 RPGs)

Funding of approved RPGs on aging: funding level—one in two

- NIA $36.5 million × 2 = $73 million (384 RPGs)
  $36.5 million additional funding (192 added RPGs)
- NIH $55.8 million × 2 = $111.6 million (588 RPGs)
  $55.8 million additional funding (294 added RPGs)
- Total $92.3 million additional funding (486 added RPGs)

These figures are estimates and may require revision as the new agenda on research is implemented. Because a significant percentage of RPG proposals represents resubmissions that were previously approved but not funded, the new funding rate for approved grants may have variable effects on the eventual number of approved grants that are reviewed for funding. Increasing the funding of approved research grants on aging should reduce the number of resubmissions that are reviewed for funding, but this trend will be offset if more investigators are encouraged by the new funding rate to resubmit grant proposals that were approved but not funded in the past. Therefore, the committee recommends that the target for funding of approved RPGs be set at one in two, subject to review and modification as the new program to expand research on aging is implemented.

Funds for age-related research sponsored by the NIA and other institutes most often support biomedical research proposals, although some funds also support research on aging in health services delivery and in social and behavioral studies. As Chapters 4 and 5 emphasize, these areas have been chronically underfunded for many years. For example, an estimated fewer than 20 percent of approved research proposals on aging in behavioral and social research are funded each year (Behavioral and Social Program, NIA).

The committee recommends that most of the funds for the behavioral and social research and health services delivery research should come from agencies that have traditionally sustained this work (e.g., Health Care Financing Administration; Alcohol, Drug Abuse, and Mental Health Administration; and the Agency for Health Care Policy and Research), and that the new funds should total at least $80 million per year in current dollars.

The 1991 NIA appropriation funds 381 RPGs (Budget Office, NIA). This new support is in concert with the committee's recommendation for increased funding of RPGs on aging, and should be extended to RPGs on aging throughout the NIH. There is information that other federal institutions may also increase their support for age-related research in the coming fiscal year.

Funding for an additional five cooperative studies on prevention, demography, epidemiology and treatment of age-related disorders is

EXECUTIVE SUMMARY AND RECOMMENDATIONS FOR FUNDING 31

recommended by the committee. These studies would implement research priorities identified earlier, and should be phased in over a 5-year period. Cooperative studies require about $5 million per study for support in current dollars (Director's Office, NIA), totaling $25 million dollars at full implementation

Funds for Training in Age-Related Studies

A recent IOM study recommended that the number of graduates in medical academic geriatric programs be increased from its current level of 100 per year to 200 to 250 per year to meet the estimated 2,100 biomedical faculty members needed in this field by the year 2000 (IOM, 1987; Rowe et al., 1987). Additional funds should be phased in over a 5-year period to implement this recommendation. Assuming that training programs for clinical investigators last 2 to 3 years, this would involve support for an additional 200 to 300 fellows in training at all levels. In addition, funds should be provided for 100 to 150 beginning clinical investigators in research on aging.

Because training programs in age-related research are currently undersubscribed, it may be best to phase in major support for training programs *after* it has been shown that the increased investment in research has attracted more students to the field. The committee believes that the current cadre of faculty members with interests in age-related research is adequate to provide initial training for increased numbers of students in this area.

The NIA estimated in 1987 that the number of trainees in age-related studies, including clinical and basic biomedical research on aging, was far short of the number needed to meet present needs (NIA, 1987). The committee recommends that steps to repair this deficiency include support for 200 additional trainees per year in basic biomedical science.

Training in behavioral and social studies and in health services delivery research has long been poorly supported (Chapters 4 and 5). In a 1987 report to Congress, the NIA predicted that more than 1,500 nonbiomedical faculty, including behavioral and social scientists, would be needed by 1990 for teaching and research needs in the field of aging, and that more than 3,500 such professionals would be needed by the year 2000 (NIA, 1987). The report noted that by 1987 only a small percentage of the 1990 training needs had been met. The committee's recommendations provide for an additional 200 doctoral trainees per year in behavioral and social studies in aging, and 140 additional trainees per year in health services delivery research.

Acknowledging that there are differences in stipends, benefits, and faculty support, depending on the level of training and the discipline involved, the committee judges that the added training across the areas of study will involve stipends, benefits, and faculty support at an average cost of $50,000 per trainee. The total number of additional trainees recommended is about 1,000, and the cost—not adjusted for inflation—for this training is $50 million per year, phased in over 5 years.

Funds for Centers

The committee recommends that funds should be phased in over the next 5 years for 10 Centers of Excellence in Research and Teaching in Geriatrics and Gerontology (Claude Pepper Centers) to be added to the current 3 NIA-sponsored Centers of Excellence.

Although the value of the centers has been questioned, and there is no clear understanding of the number of centers needed, arguments for interdisciplinary centers on aging have been given in a recent IOM report (IOM, 1987), and by the 1984 Department of Health and Human Services report on education and training in geriatrics and gerontology. According to these reports, during the early phases of the evolution of the study of aging, centers can (1) serve to mobilize and focus scarce resources, (2) provide a setting for growth of new investigators, and (3) enhance creative interaction among scientists in diverse areas of research on aging (IOM, 1987).

To merit support for the development of a Center of Excellence, "a program must meet three central goals: 1) to develop a structured, efficient training program that will attract students and produce faculty; 2) to conduct research to add to clinical knowledge, maintain an academic base, and provide role models for trainees; and 3) provide clinical care in a variety of settings. . . ." (IOM, 1987). If these goals are met and if the presence of a cadre of investigators and teachers (whose research efforts are already well supported) can be demonstrated, then a university or medical center may qualify for center support. The NIA currently supports three centers. Four additional Centers of Excellence have been approved, but not funded, and six other sites are under consideration for development. Review of applications received by the NIA indicates that sufficient faculty numbers now exist to provide the necessary professional staffing of these proposed centers (Office of the Director, NIA).

The committee believes that the new centers should be interdisciplinary in character, offering opportunities for exchange of ideas and collaboration across the fields of study of basic biomedical science, clinical research, behavioral and social studies, health services delivery, and biomedical ethics.

Estimation of the cost of the new centers is based on outlays for the Claude Pepper Geriatric Centers. These institutions required about $1.2 million per year for support (Office of Geriatrics Branch, Biomedical Research and Clinical Medicine Program, NIA). Based on this information, the 10 additional centers should cost about $12 to $15 million per year to operate (not adjusted for inflation). Funding of the new centers goes largely toward administration costs, for infrastructure costs, and toward other supports, such as salaries for beginning investigators. Direct funds for research would not depend on center support, but would come rather from grants to individual investigators and to research programs operating within the centers.

Funds for Infrastructure

Factors that make it difficult to assign costs for infrastructure research support to the different areas of research include the use of animal colonies by several disciplines for research, overlap of funds for research and infrastructure, development of databases that all disciplines may draw upon, and uncertainty in classifying new linkages to existing sources of information.

Given these constraints, the committee offers the following estimates for infrastructure costs.

Animal colonies   Based on the cost in the Pepper Centers of $375,000 per animal colony per year (Office of Geriatrics Branch, Biomedical Research and Clinical Medicine Program, NIA), not adjusted for inflation, the estimated yearly costs of animal colonies at the 10 proposed geriatric research centers are $3.75 million; adding 10 animal colonies at other university centers engaged in gerontological research brings the total cost to $7.5 million per year.

Laboratories   There are no comprehensive data on the cost of laboratories for basic biomedical and clinical research. Apart from laboratories at centers, funds are necessary to support noncenter laboratory needs in age-related basic biomedical and clinical research in other institutions. For example, three sophisticated laboratories for cell biology research to serve as regional resources for basic biomedical and clinical scientists would cost $3 million per year to staff and maintain (G.M. Martin, University of Washington, personal communication, 1989).

Databases This important infrastructure will be shared by all disciplines and consists of ongoing population studies, improved linkage to existing sources of information (e.g., Medicare data tapes), library supports such as the National Library of Medicine, and computer technology.

Research in geriatrics and gerontology will require the expansion of existing population studies (e.g., National Health and Nutrition Examination Survey) and the institution of new longitudinal demographic and epidemiological studies. The cost of such studies covers a wide range, from $1.5 million to $2.0 million per year (Office of the Director, NIA) for the Health and Retirement Study funded by the NIA, to $5 to $10 million per year (G.M. Martin, University of Washington, personal communication, 1989) for large cardiovascular prospective studies. The committee estimates that population studies would come to about $30 million per year. Another $10 million per year, shared among the disciplines, would be needed to add computer technology, to fund improved access to existing databases, and to increase the capacity of reference sources such as the National Library of Medicine.

All told, the estimated nonassigned infrastructure support totals $40 million per year. Total costs for infrastructure, not adjusted for inflation, are estimated at $50.5 million per year, phased in over 5 years.

Funds for Construction

Construction costs include those for 10 additional multidisciplinary centers and those for out-of-center animal facilities and laboratories. The cost of construction of the Mental Retardation Research Centers supported by the National Institute of Child Health and Human Development was, on average, $10 million per center; the federal government provided 75 percent of the funding, and local and state organizations made up the difference. Using these figures, with the federal government providing 75 percent of the cost of construction, the committee estimates that the total one-time cost for 10 new geriatric research centers will be $75 million, not adjusted for inflation, phased in over 5 years. Center costs include animal housing.

Additional animal housing will cost $300 to $400 per square foot (Office of Resources Development, NIA). If 10 animal facilities are built outside the centers, and if total floor space at each of these additional institutions comes to 1,000 square feet (assuming an average of 5 separate projects at each institution), total costs will be about $3.5 million. Costs to construct new laboratories, based on the committee's best estimate, are assessed at an additional $30 million, not adjusted for inflation.

The committee therefore estimates that the total one-time costs for construction, not adjusted for inflation, will be about $110 million; as described above, these costs are to be phased in over a 5-year period, with $33 million of this sum assigned to construction of infrastructure supports distributed among several areas of research.

Table 3 demonstrates the effect of low, intermediate, and full funding levels on implementation of the research agenda. For example, funding at 20 percent to 40 percent of the recommended level, phased in over 5 years, would add only about 20 to 40 age-related research projects per year, or less than 10 percent to the total number of approved and funded research project grants on aging each year. Support for trainees over 5 years at this level would add only 40 to 80 trainees per year, or 4 percent to 8 percent per year of the additional number needed. To implement research on aging in the coming decade, funding levels for resources should approach or equal the recommended total of $312 million per year, plus construction monies.

Recommendations for funding outlined in this section were based, as far as possible, on known costs for construction, infrastructure, grant support, research centers, and training. Determination of funding needs will require further examination and review prior to implementation of the new research agenda. The estimates given here represent a first step in this process.

IMPLICATIONS FOR FUNDING AGENCIES

Support for the research agenda can come from many sources. The committee suggests the following:

- Federal agency support: Support by the federal government has been detailed in the section describing funding requirements for research. As noted, large-scale projects require federal support. Additionally, the federal government should provide research funds for research in biomedical ethics. Early in this effort, the NIA and/or other agencies should convene a national conference to determine the need for support, levels of funding, and ways of implementing the research agenda on biomedical ethics.
- Private and corporate foundations: The increased flexibility of foundations makes them better able to support innovative research programs—both basic and applied—with relatively short-term goals. It would also be appropriate for foundations to join in supporting fellowships to train scientists for age-related research and to partici-

TABLE 3 Scenarios of Partial (Low, Medium, and High) Support for Aging Research

Research Support	Scenarios (in millions of dollars)		
	Low	Medium	High
Total yearly funds (% of recommended)	$62-115 (20-37%)	$156-215 (50-69%)	$250-312 (80-100%)
NIH support for RPGs (additional number per year)	$18-37 (97-194)	$46-64 (243-340)	$74-92 (389-486)
Cooperative clinical trials (additional number per year)	$5 (1)	$10-15 (2-3)	$20-25 (4-5)
Non-NIH support for behavioral/social and health services delivery research	$16-32	$40-56	$64-80
Training positions (additional number funded per year)	$10-20 (200-400)	$25-35 (500-700)	$40-50 (800-1000)
Centers of Excellence (additional number funded)	$3-6 (2-4)	$7-10 (5-7)	$12-15 (8-10)
Infrastructure	$10-20	$25-35	$40-50
Construction	$22-44	$55-80	$88-110

NOTE: Totals may not equal sums of columns because of rounding off. Funds are for yearly funding of resources, except for construction funds. Construction funds are a one-time cost. All estimates are in current dollars.

pate in the funding of geriatric research centers. Foundations can further support research in geriatrics and gerontology by funding national conferences to plan for research and dissemination of research findings or by funding training programs such as the Brookdale Foundation support of the NIA Summer Training Institute for young researchers.

• Industry support: Resources to support new technologies, evaluate

new drug therapy, and develop educational programs could be provided by industry sources.
* Combined support: Government, foundations, and industry could combine resources for nationwide policy conferences on age-related research, support for fellowships, development of geriatric research centers, and creation of functions to facilitate communication about studies in aging among different institutions. A recent IOM workshop recommended that planning be undertaken to explore and implement collaboration between government and industry in biomedical research and education (IOM, 1989).

CONCLUDING COMMENTS

The committee notes that the community of health science researchers is a great national asset—unmatched in number and productivity. Moreover, the cadre of scientists working in aging has increased rapidly throughout the country over the last 10 years and provides a major resource for new advances in basic and applied research. Prospects are bright for the application of new knowledge in the service of improved social, psychological, and physical health for older persons, for those who will reach old age in the near future, and especially for those who are now young. The numerous areas of basic and applied research in aging presently led by U.S. scientists also are a foundation for major innovation and application in the private sector. There is great potential for new drugs and consumer goods adapted to the special needs of older persons; the world market for them is growing rapidly. Moreover, the principles of genetic engineering already exist not only for organ repair and replacement but also for control of the adverse effects of inherited genes. Thus, the goals of this 20-year plan for research point to a unique U.S. role in meeting the needs of the older population throughout the world.

REFERENCES

Advisory Panel on Alzheimer's Disease. 1989. Report of the Advisory Panel on Alzheimer's Disease. DHHS Pub. No. (ADM) 89-1644. Washington, D.C.: U.S. Government Printing Office.

Baum, B. J. 1988. Oral cavity. Pp. 157-166 in Geriatric Medicine, J. W. Rowe and R. W. Besdine, eds. Boston: Little, Brown.

Berger, T. W., S. D. Berry, and R. F. Thompson. 1986. Role of the hippocampus in classical conditioning of aversive and appetitive behaviors. Pp. 203-239 in The Hippocampus, vol. 4, R. L. Isaacson and K. H. Pribam, eds. New York: Plenum.

Cummings, S. R., J. L. Kelsey, M. C. Nevitt, and K. J. O'Dowd. 1985. Epidemiology of osteoporosis and osteoporotic fractures. Epidemiology Review 7:178-190.

Diokno, A. C., B. M. Brock, M. B. Brown, and A. R. Herzog. 1986. Prevalence of urinary incontinence and other urological symptoms in the non-institutionalized elderly. Journal of Urology 136:1022-1025.
Finch, C. 1987. Environmental influences on the aging brain. Pp. 77-91 in Perspectives in Behavioral Medicine, M. W. Riley, J. Matarazzo, and A. Baum, eds. Hillsdale, N.J.: Lawrence Erlbaum Associates.
Finlayson, R. E., and L. M. Martin. 1982. Recognition and management of depression in the elderly. Mayo Clinic Proceedings 57:115-120.
Fries, J. F. 1980. Aging, natural death and the compression of morbidity. New England Journal of Medicine 303:130-135.
Fries, J. F. 1990. The sunny side of aging (editorial). Journal of the American Medical Association 263:2354-2355.
Graves, R. 1955. The Greek Myths, p. 150. Baltimore: Penguin Books.
Gruenberg, E. M. 1977. The failures of success. Milbank Memorial Fund Quarterly; Health and Society 55:3-24.
Hagnell, O., J. Lanke, B. Rorsman, R. Ohman, and L. Ojesjö. 1983. Current trends in the incidence of senile and multi-infarct dementia. Archives of Psychiatry and Neurological Science 233:423.
Institute of Medicine. 1987. Academic geriatrics for the year 2000 (report of the Committee on Leadership for Academic Geriatric Medicine). Journal of the American Geriatrics Society 35:773-791.
Institute of Medicine. 1989. Report of a Workshop. Government and Industry Collaboration in Biomedical Research and Education. Washington, D.C.: National Academy Press.
Jensen, T. S., I. K. Genefke, N. Hyldebrandt, H. Pedersen, H. D. Petersen, and B. Weile. 1982. Cerebral atrophy in young torture victims. New England Journal of Medicine 307:1341-1344.
Kane, R., D. Solomon, J. Beck, E. Keeler, and R. Kane. 1980. The future need for geriatric manpower in the United States. New England Journal of Medicine 302:1327-1332.
Katz, S., L. G. Branch, M. H. J. Branson, J. A. Papsidero, J. C. Beck, and D. S. Greer. 1983. Active life expectancy. New England Journal of Medicine 309:1218-1224.
Lipowski, Z. J. 1989. Delirium in the elderly patient. New England Journal of Medicine 320:578-582.
Manton, K. G., and B. J. Soldo. 1985. Dynamics of health changes in the oldest old: Perspectives and evidence. Milbank Memorial Fund Quarterly; Health and Society 63:206-285.
Martin, G. M. 1979. Proliferative homeostasis and its age-related aberrations. Mechanisms of Aging and Development 9:385-391.
Movsesian, M. A. 1990. Effect on physician-scientists of the low funding rate of NIH grant applications. New England Journal of Medicine 322:1602-1604.
National Center for Health Statistics. 1985. National Health Interview Survey. Vital and Health Statistics, Series 10, No. 150. DHHS Pub. No. (PHS) 85-1578. Washington, D.C.: U.S. Government Printing Office.
National Center for Health Statistics. 1987. Health Statistics on Older Persons, United States 1986. Vital and Health Statistics, Series 3, No. 25, 1987, pp. 41-55. Washington, D.C.: U.S. Government Printing Office.
National Center for Health Statistics. 1988. Current estimates for the national health interview survey: U.S., 1, 1987. Vital and Health Statistics, Series 10, No. 166, DHHS Pub. No. 88-1594. Washington, D.C: U.S. Government Printing Office.

EXECUTIVE SUMMARY AND RECOMMENDATIONS FOR FUNDING 39

National Center for Health Statistics. 1989. Vital and Health Statistics Report, No. 173 and 37, No. 5, Supplement. Washington, D.C.: U.S. Government Printing Office.

National Institute on Aging. 1978. Our Future Selves. Bethesda, Md.: U.S. Government Printing Office.

National Institute on Aging. 1982. Toward an Independent Old Age: A National Plan for Research on Aging. Bethesda, Md.: U.S. Government Printing Office.

National Institute on Aging. 1987. Personnel for Health Needs of the Elderly Through Year 2020, p. 3. Administrative Document, U.S. Department of Health and Human Services. Washington, D.C.: U.S. Government Printing Office.

Ouslander, J. G., R. L. Kane, and I. B. Abrass. 1982. Urinary incontinence in elderly nursing home patients. Journal of the American Medical Association 248:1194.

Pepper Commission. 1990. A Call for Action: Final Report of the Pepper Commission on Comprehensive Care. Washington, D.C.: U.S. Government Printing Office.

Reuben, D. B., T. B. Bradley, J. Zwanziger, J. H. Hirsh, and J. C. Beck. 1990. Candidates for the certificate of added qualifications in geriatric medicine. Who, why and when? Journal of the American Geriatrics Society 38:483-488.

Rice, D. 1989. Demographics and Health of the Elderly: Past Trends and Projections. Report to the Prospective Payment Advisory Committee. Washington, D.C.: Prospective Payment Advisory Committee.

Rowe, J. W., E. Grossman, and E. Bond. 1987. Academic geriatrics for the year 2000: An Institute of Medicine report. New England Journal of Medicine 316:1425-1428.

Schneider, E. L., and J. M. Guralnick. 1990. The aging of America. Impact on health care costs. Journal of the American Medical Association 263:2335-2340.

Select Committee on Aging, U.S. House of Representatives. 1985. America's Elderly at Risk. Committee Publication No. 99-508. Washington, D.C.: U.S. Government Printing Office.

Select Committee on Aging, U.S. House of Representatives. 1990. Emptying the Elderly's Pocketbook—Growing Impact of Rising Health Costs. Committee Publication No. 101-746. Washington D.C.: U.S. Government Printing Office.

Soldo, B. J., and K. G. Manton. 1988. Demography: Characteristics and implications of an aging population. Pp. 12-22 in Geriatric Medicine, J. W. Rowe and R. W. Besdine, eds. Boston: Little, Brown.

U.S. Bureau of the Census. 1984. Projections of the population of the United States by age, sex, and race: 1988 to 2080. Current Population Reports, Series P-25, No. 1,018. Washington, D.C.: U.S. Government Printing Office.

Waldo, D. R., S. T. Sonnefeld, D. R. McKusick, and R. H. Arnett. 1989. Health expenditures by age group, 1977 and 1987. Health Care Financing Review 10:111-120.

Weiler, P. G. 1987. The public health impact of Alzheimer's disease. American Journal of Public Health 77:1157-1158.

World Health Organization. 1982. World Program of Action Concerning Disabled Persons. Geneva: World Health Organization.

1

Introduction

Over the past two decades the American system of health care and the biomedical, social, and behavioral sciences have begun to come to grips with the overwhelming consequences of the rapid and dramatic growth of the elderly population. Long neglected, the topic of aging has attracted substantial attention as this country seeks to build the infrastructure of a national research and academic capacity in aging. For instance, the National Institute on Aging (NIA) and scores of university and medical school academic programs in gerontology and geriatrics have been established, and recently developed training programs are generating a cadre of sophisticated gerontologists and geriatricians.

In addition to building the foundation for what is becoming one of the nation's major new scientific efforts, recent financial investments in aging have already yielded important research findings across a spectrum of inquiry, including the basic mechanisms of aging, the physiology of normal aging, the social and behavioral aspects of aging, health services research for older persons, and the etiology and management of age-related disease. A bibliometric search, conducted in conjunction with the project that forms the basis of this report, shows that between 1983 and 1987, taking into account overall growth in research, there was a 70 percent relative increase in scholarly publications in aging. Although growth in some of these areas, particularly in age-related disease (e.g., Alzheimer's disease), has clearly outstripped growth in other areas, all domains have seen substantial growth from their meager beginnings over four decades ago.

Notwithstanding this progress, the medical and scientific community's knowledge, research, and clinical capacity lag far behind the human need, and society currently is paying a heavy price for decades of neglect of aging and the special needs of older persons. The burgeoning elderly population will increasingly burden the nation's fiscally troubled health care system. Despite our recognition that investments in research ultimately yield substantial financial, clinical, and social benefits, the nation's commitment to aging research is minuscule in comparison to the costs of health care for older persons. Even in the case of Alzheimer's disease—one of the best-supported areas of age-related research—expenditures for scientific investigation equal less than one-half of one percent (0.1 percent) of the costs of care for the victims of this disease (Report of the Advisory Panel on Alzheimer's Disease 1988-1989, U.S. Department of Health and Human Services, DHHS Pub. No. (ADM)89-1644).

Given the heavy toll and long duration of chronic illness and disability, the small national commitment to aging research is a particularly risky and potentially wasteful strategy, especially in light of the enormous promise of properly supported research, not only to improve the status of older adults, but also to reduce substantially the costs of their care. Effective strategies against many disorders common in old age, such as dementia, urinary incontinence, osteoporosis, and falls, could yield huge financial savings and, at the same time, enhance well-being. Likewise, research is needed on intervention strategies to ameliorate the deleterious conditions of economic and social dependency, the growing caregiving burden, and inadequate coping capacities. Such research could reduce negative health effects and their attendant costs while improving the aging experience for millions of Americans.

A factor limiting the development of gerontologic and geriatric research is the critical shortage of workers in this area. Current funding mechanisms often do not provide adequate research or training support for young investigators interested in studying aspects of aging. The United States must develop effective mechanisms to attract established scientists from other fields into aging or age-related research, and it must construct attractive career ladders for young investigators from a variety of fields who enter the study of aging as a career.

A growing sense of urgency mandates that the time is right to narrow the gap between the needs of an aging society and the scientific knowledge base. Building on the existing academic substrata, the medical and scientific community can leverage both new knowledge and tools from other fields to develop aging research into a mature component of the national scientific portfolio. For example, dramatic recent developments in several fields—from molecular biology to the social sciences—await application to age-related issues and hold the potential of rapidly advancing the nascent fields of gerontology and geriatrics. There is an increasing awareness that the field of aging may be entering a phase of major breakthroughs that have the potential not only of increasing our understanding of age-related diseases and enhancing functions in the elderly but also, quite possibly, of beginning to solve the mystery of the human lifespan. This opportunity is constrained, however, by increasing fiscal pressures.

At this critical juncture the nation's needs demand a comprehensive plan for research on aging. This document represents the result of the Institute of Medicine's (IOM's) effort to develop a plan in recognition of this need at the request of a number of federal agencies and foundations.

The IOM convened 87 experts from various fields relevant to aging and age-related research in a two-year study to identify the needs and opportunities for research on aging in basic biomedical science, social and behavioral sciences, clinical medicine, health services delivery, and biomedical ethics. The group sought to document and outline recent exciting developments in aging research, to set clear priorities for future research, and to estimate the resources required to enter into such an agenda for the nation's research scientists. A major thrust of this report examines processes of discovery and treatment that will improve *function* in the elderly population, without denying the importance of research whose focus is restricted to investigation of disease.

This study includes three stages. During the first stage, commissioned papers were developed, and a detailed bibliometric analysis of aging research was conducted. In the second stage the expert committee met several times to deliberate and prepare this report. For the report the committee sought input from a wide variety of agencies and organizations interested in or supportive of research on aging. The committee has reviewed the current funding inventory as well as the results of the bibliometric analysis. Liaison teams comprised of experts in the areas of biomedical, clinical, behavioral and social, and health services delivery research were charged with developing a prioritized list of special research opportunities and needs for the next 10 to 20 years. In addition, two national authorities in the field of biomedical ethics provided information about research needs in this area.

After reviewing and discussing the reports of the liaison teams and ethicists, the committee sculpted the overall research agenda. Special efforts were made to identify a clear set of priorities that reflected both promising and neglected areas of inquiry rather than merely providing a compendium of current or needed research in aging. Particular attention was paid to identification of areas of age-related research that should be supported by the federal government as well as those areas that deserve the attention and support of private foundations.

In the final or third stage of this effort, the IOM will work to bring the report to the attention of policymakers, the scientific community, and the general public.

The National Research Agenda on Aging builds on two previous documents developed by the NIA—a 1978 report, *Our Future Selves*, and a 1982 report, *Toward an Independent Old Age: A National Plan for Research on Aging*—which, taken together, provided an excellent point of departure for the present work. Another major resource was an inventory of federal research on aging, compiled in 1982 by a task force of the U.S. Department of Health and Human Services.

The IOM is uniquely qualified to develop this national research agenda on aging. Since its inception in 1970 as a branch of the National Academy of Sciences, one aspect of the IOM's mission has been to advance and protect the health of the public. Several efforts over the past decade have established the IOM as an important national resource for the analysis of health policy issues on aging. These reports include (1) *Aging in Medical Education* (1978), (2) *Health in an Older Society* (1985), (3) *Improving the Quality of Care in Nursing Homes* (1986), (4) *Productive Roles in an Older Society* (1986), (5) *Academic Geriatrics for the Year 2000* (1987), and (6) *The Social and Built Environment in an Older Society* (1988). The effectiveness of the IOM in influencing public policy is evidenced by the fact that the reports on nursing home care and on academic geriatrics recently led to adoption of federal legislation implementing IOM recommendations.

In concluding this analysis, the IOM drew on special strengths: the voluntary nature of the experts' participation in IOM efforts; IOM's reputation for objectivity; its interdisciplinary membership and perspectives; its collaborative interaction with other components of the National Academy of Sciences; and the thorough, robust, and careful review of all reports prior to their release.

The committee applied important criteria in prioritizing research areas during its deliberations on this project. To qualify for consideration for a prominent place on the National Research Agenda on Aging, the area of research must have fallen within one or more of the following general categories:

- General aging processes: Such studies focus on theories of aging (diverse mechanisms of aging processes, including genetic and environmental components and their interaction) functioning at the molecular, cellular, organ, organ system, organism, and wider psychosocial and sociocultural levels.
- Important age-related disease: This might be a disease occurring predominantly in aged populations or a disease found across the lifespan whose occurrence in old age is associated with specific alterations in its presentation, course, or sequelae (e.g., diabetes).
- Factors influencing age-disease interaction: A number of lifestyle and socioenvironmental factors have an important influence both on the emergence of disease in aging populations and on the mode of presentation by the older victims of disease.
- The functional capacity of the elderly: The enormous importance of functional capacity as a determinant of the care needs of older persons dictates a special focus on those factors that limit the activity of elderly individuals and impair their independence.
- The feasibility and timeliness of the research: The committee was sensitive to the fact that "pie-in-the-sky" research agendas must be avoided in favor of feasible research, that is, research whose "time has come." Similarly, an overly conservative research strategy must be avoided since major breakthroughs often are made when special, timely windows of opportunity present themselves.

Other criteria for areas of research included their potential to (1) enhance research in other areas, as in basic studies on proliferative capacity of cells to improve studies on carcinogenesis; (2) reduce morbidity and mortality in older persons; (3) decrease costs of care; (4) increase knowledge of behavioral and social factors in health and disease; and (5) improve pharmacological treatment of patients.

During its deliberations, the committee identified 11 emerging and overarching themes relevant to the entire spectrum of research on aging. These provide a context for the consideration of the individual research areas discussed in the ensuing chapters.

1. An interdisciplinary approach to studies of aging: Many of the most intractable problems in aging research, particularly in the clinical, social, and behavioral arenas, can be properly addressed only by an interdisciplinary group. Interdisciplinary work is costly and

INTRODUCTION

often more difficult to design and conduct successfully than unidisciplinary research.

2. Increasing the body of data based on longitudinal studies: Much of the available information on aging is based on crosscohort studies that compare individuals of different age groups. Although these studies provide some perspective on the effects of aging, they are subject to a number of non-age-related influences, such as secular and cohort effects. Longitudinal studies in which serial prospective measures are made on the same individuals over time provide a much more robust approach to gerontologic and geriatric research. Longitudinal studies, although inherently more time-consuming and expensive than crosscohort studies, are relevant to all domains of research—from basic science through clinical investigation to health services research.

3. Developing research resources—databases, well-defined study populations, cell lines, animal colonies, and animal models for research on aging: Such research resources often can be used by many different investigators conducting various studies at the same time. Federal and, in some cases, foundation funds can be brought to bear to establish such resources. Increasing attention must be given to the types of resources needed to promote the development of aging research to its next level of accomplishment.

4. Areas of neglect—gender, race, cultural background, and ethnicity: Substantial increases in research on aging in members of different racial, cultural, and ethnic groups are needed to clarify the mechanisms underlying differences in the presentation, course, and sequelae of a variety of geriatric-related disorders. Additionally, gender has been shown to have a major influence on biological as well as social and behavioral aspects of aging.

5. Importance of a life-course perspective: Substantial disability and health care expenditures in old age are rooted in the lifestyle, environmental, and other psychosocial factors that begin during youth or middle age. A developmental life-course perspective should be increasingly incorporated into aging research.

6. Emphasis on studying basic mechanisms of aging: Throughout its first phase of development, most gerontologic and geriatric research was descriptive in nature. Studies of the mechanisms of age-related alterations that build on this information and the expanded application of the new and powerful investigative techniques now available are needed.

7. Specialized health promotion and disease prevention research in older populations: A revolutionary increase in life expectancy has occurred already. A corresponding increase in *active* life expectancy

or health span should be the focus of much of the next phase of aging research. Such an effort must avoid the simple generalization of health promotion/disease prevention research in middle age to older populations. Instead, it should take into account the special physiological characteristics of the elderly and should focus in particular on such disorders as dementia, incontinence, and falls, which are particularly common and disabling in elderly populations.

8. Studies of the role of genetics, social, and environmental factors as modifiers of aging: The effects of the aging process itself have been exaggerated; the modifying effects of the individual's genetic background, nutritional status, exercise, personal habits, and psychosocial factors have been underestimated.

9. The psychological and sociological context of the individual: Interdisciplinary approaches that consider both the influence of the individual's behavior and environment and social interactions and support systems will be crucial. Equally important is the need to explain specific age-related findings.

10. Expansion of health services delivery research: Many of the issues discussed in this section (e.g., the study of the effectiveness of interventions and the investigation of financing of care) may be implemented by the techniques and mechanisms special to the field of health services delivery. This discipline often serves as the interface between scientific application and political policy decisions affecting the delivery of health care to millions of Americans. Health services delivery research can provide objective information to policymakers, assisting them in developing their programs on a more scientific basis and providing tools for analyzing the usefulness of these programs.

11. Ethical considerations in the care of the elderly as a research focus: Previous agendas for research on aging have seriously neglected ethical issues, such as the rationing of health care and the provision of care to and the conduct of research on demented and irreversibly ill older persons, especially with regard to the application of life-sustaining technologies.

One of the major scientific challenges for the United States over the next decade will be to enlarge our research capacity in aging so that we gain the knowledge necessary to deal with the health, social, and psychological needs of a rapidly aging society. This plan provides a prioritized and rational blueprint for that research development.

2

Basic Biomedical Research

The term *aging* can refer to changes taking place during any stage of life. Some of these changes are benign, with no evident adverse effects; others are eventually harmful. The dysfunctional changes associated with accelerated mortality rates during the later phase of adult life are collectively called senescence. Senescence is associated both with diseases of specific organs and tissues and with diffuse disorders that defy conventional classification. Within the vast scope of these phenomena of aging, many of the problems of senescence can be explored scientifically. Continued research not only will yield new interventions into specific disorders of senescence but also will lead to the discovery of the nature of many basic biological mechanisms that change during the aging process.

A number of puzzling questions about aging have attracted the interest of biomedical researchers. Why, for example, do humans differ so individually in aging changes of bone, brain, and heart? Here we see how genetic and epigenetic factors produce different responses to environmental influences throughout the lifespan. Because the environment begins to influence the organism long before birth, aging represents an array of processes that develop over the entire lifespan. Thus, environmental influences on genetic and epigenetic characteristics of an individual may give rise to preconditions of disability and disability itself long before senescence is manifested. The potential for reversing or delaying disability depends on the still unknown nature and extent of fundamental changes in gene expression through the aging process. Careful study of environmental-genetic interactions throughout life is required.

Clearly, aging is a unique frontier of the life sciences that requires examination by a wide array of scientific disciplines. Research in aging will clarify the basis of many specific disorders of human aging and, in so doing, will add to the proud advances that have eliminated so many diseases of children and younger adults. Moreover, the ability to understand aging requires a powerful intellectual synthesis of diverse research areas that presently stand apart from each other because of their historical focus on specific organs and diseases.

Fundamental information about the basic mechanisms of aging still is woefully inadequate. Critically necessary is aging research in the basic disciplines of biology: genetics, biochemistry, cell biology, neurobiology, developmental biology, and others. The history of science amply demonstrates that major advances often come from serendipitous discoveries. Thus, in any agenda designed to establish priorities and to estimate the resources for aging research, it is of utmost importance that investigator-initiated research be protected. This should provide the core from which many major concepts and discoveries will emerge.

Research on basic cellular functions has brought many new insights into the biological mechanisms of aging (Röhme, 1981; Stanulis-Praeger, 1981) and research gives ample reason for optimism. Equally, new, improved, and expanded model systems for the study of aging have been uncovered; these include rodents from food-restricted colonies with enhanced lifespans and delayed, reduced, or absent age-related pathologies (Masoro, 1988); methods for the creation of strains of laboratory mice with a wide array of targeted mutations (selection of substrains with specific genetic characteristics); breeding lines of unusually long-lived insects from genetically heterogeneous stocks (Dice and Goff, 1987); and identification of a single gene mutation that increases lifespan in the nematode *Caenorhabditis elegans*. Progress has been made in the development of chemically defined media for cultivation of normal diploid somatic cells to facilitate analysis of mechanisms of clonal senescence and cellular repair.

Major conceptual and methodological advances in the techniques of molecular biology, especially in molecular genetics, are leading to an increased understanding of gene expression at the molecular level. Genetic maps are reaching high resolutions (markers at about one million nucleotide base pairs), with the potential for mapping and cloning the dominant genes responsible for such various age-related disorders as familial Alzheimer's disease (St. George-Hyslop et al., 1987).

Finally, scientists are increasingly aware of the intellectual challenges posed by biogerontology as a major uncharted frontier of biology.

The committee believes that elucidation of the biological mechanisms of aging is an achievable goal. The major recommendations that follow focus attention on a broad array of important areas of investigation that are both feasible and critical to our knowledge of aging and its basic processes.

Three main criteria were utilized in the selection of the research priorities in the field of basic biomedical investigation:

1. Feasibility of the research in the context of current advances in the biological sciences: Enough is known to permit immediate expansion of existing efforts in these areas and to plan for and develop the resources needed during the next decade. Expansion of these research areas will have an immediate impact on the understanding of a number of aspects of the aging process.

2. Importance of these research areas insofar as potential findings can be applied to the treatment of major disabilities of later life: In the examples discussed, the committee believes that biomedical research eventually will lead to prevention of these disorders.

3. Potential of the research areas selected to catalyze a cascade of productivity in many other areas of health research, including areas outside of aging that share technology or concepts with gerontology.

RESEARCH PRIORITIES

- **The committee proposes a major new initiative to achieve understanding of the basis for the pervasive disturbances in the regulation of proliferative homeostasis that accompany aging in essentially all animals, including humans.**

These disturbances in proliferative homeostasis, a fundamental process responsible for appropriate replacement of cells that have become lost either because of exposure to toxins or because of endogenous physiological processes, play major roles in cellular regeneration and repair and in the genesis of several of the most important age-related human disorders: cancer, atherosclerosis, osteoarthritis, benign prostatic hyperplasia, and altered immune function (Martin, 1979). This new major national initiative should be comparable in emphasis and scope to the NIA's highest research priority—Alzheimer's disease and the neurobiology of aging.

- The second priority research recommendation is that basic research in the neurosciences (including the peripheral and central nervous systems) and the current special research initiatives on Alzheimer's disease should be continued and expanded.

Funding allocations for the foregoing should supplement, not supplant, existing research support and should not detract from other areas of investigation. Fundamental studies on aging and the regulation of gene expression and macromolecular syntheses, postsynthetic modifications of proteins and protein degradation, membrane changes, and other fundamental research approaches are essential to the studies envisioned above and to all facets of biomedical exploration. To achieve the above-noted research goals, major new research resources are required for direct support of research projects, additional training programs, expansion of current centers devoted to studies on aging, and enlargement of the current infrastructure for basic biomedical scientific exploration. These are described later in this chapter.

ADDITIONAL RESEARCH OPPORTUNITIES

The identification of two major research recommendations in no way is intended to detract from the importance of other areas of biogerontological research. Some promising research directions not included in the major recommendations also are worthy of encouragement and support. A brief discussion of some of these important research directions follows.

Although one major emphasis of this report is on proliferating cells, the role of nondividing cell types in the process of aging should be explored further. These studies should focus on postmitotic cells, such as neurons and cardiac and skeletal muscle cells, as well as on conditionally proliferating cells, such as hepatocytes (Martin, 1977), and will provide important information about aging mechanisms that have been neglected. Presently, little or no information is available about repair and regeneration in these cells. For example, does macromolecular turnover change with age? How are cell surface properties altered? Do signal transduction mechanisms change?

Another area of emphasis is that of systems physiology. Most gerontologists agree that aging is a multifactorial process, involving many cells, tissues, and organ types. Research must be carried out on the major integrative systems in physiology. The effects of aging on the endocrine/neuroendocrine and immune systems (Finch et al.,

1985; Miller, 1990) must be understood if we are to understand the organism's aging phenotype. Dietary restriction as a modulator of lifespan in rats and mice represents an important probe for understanding aging changes (Masoro, 1988). Similarly, regulation of reproductive physiology and of the developmental process in general represents a potentially important analogue for the aging process and should be emphasized (Finch et al., 1985).

The fact that cells, tissues, and organs do not age at the same rate among species or even among individuals within a species poses a key complicating factor for these studies. Hepatocytes, for example, may be functionally youthful in an individual whose nervous system or cardiac function is seriously impaired as a result of aging or disease. The use of lifespan as an end point for aging has further hampered the interpretation of numerous studies. The field sorely needs measures of senescence based on functional capacity. Thus, descriptive studies of each system, evaluated in relation to overall functional competence and mortality risk, are critical to the development of meaningful biomarkers for aging, and for the identification of dysfunctional aging (senescence). Such biomarkers would increase scientific understanding of the factors that influence the rate of aging along the continuum of biological change and would contribute to the development of interventions that might delay or reverse dysfunctional aging (senescence). The concept of biomarkers applies at many levels, from cellular biology to the more complex interactions that are the object of scientific study in clinical, behavioral and social, and other areas of health care research (Sprott and Baker, 1988).

Abundant evidence is available of the accumulation of abnormal proteins during the course of aging and in the development of age-related diseases, such as the neurofibrillary tangles and beta-amyloid of Alzheimer's disease (Stadtman, 1988). Moreover, many tissues acquire inactive enzymes during aging (Dice and Goff, 1987). A major question concerns the pathogenesis of such abnormal proteins. The general question of altered gene expression in aging is of the utmost urgency if we are to understand the biological bases of aging, and the role of environmental influences, such as free radicals, radiation, and various toxicants, raises an additional and pressing set of questions about how the environment may influence aging (Ames et al., 1985).

While some research is focusing on various types of molecular damage, studies on the mechanisms of selective changes in gene activity should receive special emphasis. The powerful tools of recombinant DNA genetics are being applied to these questions. For

Ten additional Centers of Excellence in Research and Education in Geriatrics and Gerontology (Claude Pepper Centers) should be established to maintain the foregoing resources. Also to be developed is resource support to perform high-technology tasks, such as specialized laboratories for cell biology, that are fundamental to a wide range of aging research. Three such laboratories are recommended to serve as regional infrastructure support for basic biomedical studies on aging.

There is evidence that the absence of sufficient laboratory space has been a major impediment to more rapid progress in Alzheimer's disease research. Congress can address this problem, in part, by appropriating construction funds already authorized by legislation creating Alzheimer's Disease Research Centers.

In addition, we need to produce at least 200 more well-trained research scientists per year with commitments to research on aging. To the aggressive pursuit of young researchers by existing training programs should be added new programs designed specifically to recruit scientists with established reputations in other fields.

In view of the special nature of gerontological research, the committee strongly recommends that mechanisms for long-term research and research training support (5 to 7 years) become more widely available.

New funding for research is required to implement these initiatives. Further sums will be needed for training, infrastructure support, and construction and renovation to house the research resources in the field. In addition, the basic biomedical research program will share in the development of additional multidisciplinary centers for research and education (Claude Pepper Centers) and in the support of infrastructure resources (e.g., computer capability; data banks, including population studies; and library support).

With additional support for research grants, infrastructure, and centers, a significant increase should follow both in the number of investigators who turn their attention to the phenomena of aging and in a stepped-up intensity in the nature of the research currently under way. Increased support for research careers in the study of aging should also lead to greater enrollment of young professionals in those training programs now undersubscribed. Both cancer biologists and gerontologists are now well aware of the close interrelationships in the regulation of senescence and neoplasia.

The expanded effort proposed in this report can be expected to lead to an increased understanding of the nature of cell regulation and how changes in this process lead to those diseases of aging characterized by aberrant proliferation, such as cancer, atherosclerosis, osteoarthritis, and prostatic hypertrophy. In addition, understanding the genetic and epigenetic regulation of functional capacity as manifested at the cellular level will provide models to understand senescence and its regulation in a wide variety of cell and tissue types. Insight into these regulatory factors will yield substantial dividends in terms of the prevention of and therapy for the illnesses and disabilities of older individuals.

CROSSCUTTING ISSUES

Biomedical research has only recently begun to examine the role of gender, race, and ethnic background and the relevance of those issues to altered trajectories of aging. The gender differential in lifespan is one fundamental issue that needs clarification. In developed countries, for example, females enjoy a substantially greater average lifespan. Although a major reason for this difference perhaps can be attributed to lifestyle differences (smoking, alcohol, violence, and fat ingestion), other reasons for the female lifespan advantage are obscure. For other mammalian species it is still not clear whether a consistent gender differential in lifespan really exists. In any case, sociobehavioral factors perhaps are crucial in these effects and in the gender differential in the incidence of many age-related disorders.

Another crosscutting issue is that of ethics. What are the ethical considerations in doing basic biomedical research? What about the ethical questions attendant upon genetic engineering? In 1990 human gene transplants became a reality. What are the ethics concerning those gene transplants that might prevent the development of age-related dysfunctions but that might as well have adverse effects on younger individuals?

Finally, there is and will continue to be a need for regularly updated interdisciplinary education, which should be developed at several levels of sophistication and targeted for a range of professional specialization in health caregiving and administration.

REFERENCES

Ames, B. N., R. L. Saul, E. Schwiers, R. Adelman, and R. Cathcart. 1985. Oxidative DNA damages related to cancer and aging: Assay of thymine glycol, thymidine glycol, and hydroxymethyluracil in human and rat urine. Pp. 137-144 in Molecular Biology of Aging: Gene Stability and Gene Expression, R. S. Sohal, L. S. Birnbaum, and R. G. Cutler, eds. New York: Raven Press.

Dice, J. F., and S. A. Goff. 1987. Error catastrophe and aging: Future directions of research. Pp. 155-168 in Modern Biological Theories of Aging, H. R. Warner, R. N. Butler, R. L. Sprott, and E. L. Schneider, eds. New York: Raven Press.

Finch, C., L. S. Felicio, C. V. Mobbs, and J. F. Nelson. 1985. Ovarian and steroidal influences on neuroendocrine aging processes in female rodents. Endocrinology Review 5:467-497.

Martin, G. M. 1977. Cellular aging—Postreplicative cells. Review (Part 2). American Journal of Pathology 89:513-530.

Martin, G. M. 1979. Proliferative homeostasis and its age-related aberrations. Mechanisms of Aging and Development 9:385-391.

Masoro, E. J. 1988. Minireview. Food restriction in rodents: An evaluation of its role in the study of aging. Journal of Gerontology: Biological Sciences 43:1359-1364.

Miller, R. 1990. Aging and the Immune Response. Pp. 157-180 in Handbook of the Biology of Aging, E. Schneider and J. W. Rowe, eds. New York: Academic Press.

Röhme, D. 1981. Evidence for a relationship between longevity of mammalian species and life spans of normal fibroblasts in vitro and erythrocytes in vivo. Proceedings of the National Academy of Sciences U.S.A. 78:5009-5013.

Sprott, R. L, and G. T. Baker III, eds. 1988. Special Issue: Biomarkers of Aging. Experimental Gerontology, vol. 23.

Stadtman, E. R. 1988. Protein modification imaging. Journal of Gerontology 43:B112-B120.

Stanulis-Praeger, B. M. 1981. Cellular senescence revisited: A review. Mechanisms of Aging and Development 38:1-48.

St. George-Hyslop, P. H., R. E. Tanzi, R. J. Polinsky, J. L. Haines, L. Nee, P. C. Watkins, R. H. Myers, R. G. Feldman, D. Pollen, D. Drachman, J. Growdon, A. Bruni, J. F. Concin, D. Salmon, P. Frommelt, L. Amaducci, S. Sorbi, S. Piacentine, G. D. Stewart, W. J. Hobbs, P. M. Conneally, and J. F. Gusella. 1987. The genetic defect causing familial Alzheimer's disease maps on chromosome 21. Science 235:885-890.

Verdonik, F., and L. R. Sherrod. 1984. An Inventory of Longitudinal Research on Childhood and Adolescence. New York: Social Science Research Council.

3

Clinical Research

The rapid growth of clinical research in geriatric medicine over the past decade permits a broad-based attack on myriad important and previously neglected research questions across several research areas. These include investigations of age-dependent changes in an array of physiologic systems, pathophysiology and management of a number of diseases relevant to aging populations, and characterization of the problems of frail, elderly people, including those in long-term care facilities.

Building on the impressive though unsystematic database that has been developed, a consensus is emerging regarding the most important lines of future research inquiry. That consensus, sharpened by the systematic discussions involved in preparing this National Research Agenda, focuses on two key areas that can serve as the basis for specific research questions and proposals: (1) research into the causes, prevention, management, and rehabilitation of disability in older persons, including a focus on geriatric syndromes; and (2) studies of age-dependent physiologic change and specific pathologic entities.

Recommendations for specific studies within these two major topic areas overlap significantly, reflecting both the multifactorial nature of disease and disability in old age and the absence of clear, common pathways of declining function in older people. Such overlap also is inherent in the area of clinical research since the field ranges from molecular biology and genetics to epidemiology, and draws on information supplied by basic biomedical research, health services studies, and the behavioral and social sciences. Clinical research shares many techniques and subjects with other areas of investigation but has a special focus on the connections between organic illness and functional status and on specific interventions to treat or prevent organic diseases. Several recent Institute of Medicine (IOM) studies on research into the effectiveness and outcomes of health care have described the potential for interaction between clinical research and other areas of investigation in the study of older patients (IOM, 1989, 1990a).

In addition to overlapping with other areas of research, the clinical research priorities described below share a common opportunity for investigation—study of the value of rehabilitative care in clinical outcomes, in cost benefits, and in cost effectiveness.

RESEARCH PRIORITIES

- **The first priority is research into the causes, prevention, management, and rehabilitation of functional disability in elderly persons.**

The overwhelming importance of functional capacity as a determinant of older persons' needs dictates a special focus on factors that limit the independence of elderly individuals. Increasingly, the clinical geriatric research community recognizes and agrees that it is well positioned to make significant short-term advances in the understanding of the physiologic and pathophysiologic mechanisms underlying the dependency and frailty that characterize the final stages of life.

Although at any given time, a majority of older persons are free of significant disability, the rate of disability rises with age. The National Health Interview Survey (National Center for Health Statistics, 1985) reported that 23 percent of all elderly persons are unable to perform at least one of the activities of daily living (ADLs). These ADLs include bathing, dressing, grooming, going to the toilet, being able to move from bed to chair, being continent, and being able to feed oneself. About half of those 85 years of age and older need assistance to perform one or more ADLs or to carry out one or more instrumental activities of daily living (IADLs). These include shopping, using public transportation, cooking, using the telephone, housekeeping, and managing finances (Dawson et al., 1987). In order for an older person to be independent, he or she must be able to perform these activities. Clearly, with increasing inability to perform ADLs and IADLs, one's dependency on others for care increases. As many as one to one-and-a-half million elderly individuals residing in the community or in institutions are unable to carry out five or more ADLs (Branch et al., 1984). However, recent studies indicate that such deficits are not static and may indeed respond to rehabilitation (Williams, 1988).

Within the general area of functional disability research, two general areas stand out: studies of health promotion and disease prevention in older persons and studies of specific geriatric syndromes.

Health Promotion and Disease Prevention in Old Age

The mechanisms and diseases that lead to age-related increases in disability have not been elucidated. With few exceptions, research in health promotion and disease prevention has not focused on older cohorts. Although substantial data on the relationship of traditional cardiovascular risk factors to the subsequent incidence of cardiovascular disease in older men and women are emerging from the aging Framingham cohorts, few data are available to indicate whether intervention in these risk factors affects subsequent rates of cardiovascular disease, including stroke, heart attacks, and congestive heart failure. Some limited data exist in the area of diastolic hypertension, and a major multicenter study is under way to evaluate the contributions of isolated elevations in systolic blood pressure to these end points, particularly stroke. However, few studies adequately address remediable risk factors for other important geriatric disorders, including osteoporosis, dementia, disability, and total mortality.

Too often, investigators have generalized findings from middle-aged adults to older individuals without recognizing the major effects of the substantially altered physiologic substrates with advancing age. No a priori assumption can be made that risk factors for important diseases in middle age carry the same relative or the same attributable risk in old age. From a lifespan perspective, it is important to note that many prevention issues pertinent to older people should first be addressed to young adults (IOM, 1990a,b).

While a substantial number of specific research areas have been identified, two are particularly salient:

1. Research should be conducted on the interacting effects of age, lifestyle factors, and disease on the disability status of older persons.

2. Studies should be undertaken to determine the effectiveness of various disease prevention strategies or practices in older persons.

Studies of Geriatric Syndromes

While functional disability may be the final common pathway of frailty for many older individuals, the specific clinical manifestations of disability vary among individuals. In many patients functional dependence is associated with the emergence of one or several specific geriatric clinical syndromes that may share some basic underlying pathophysiologic mechanisms. Geriatric syndromes represent a cluster of symptoms, conditions, and disabilities resulting in a variety of physiologic changes, pathologic conditions, comorbid conditions, and environmental challenges.

These disorders are quite common in persons over age 75 and result in substantial disability, morbidity, and decreased quality of life. A number of these syndromes—including failure to thrive; impaired postural stability, strength, and mobility; mismanagement of medications; urinary incontinence; and delirium—have been neglected for some time but are particularly ripe for major research advances.

Failure to Thrive (Inanition)

This is a syndrome of weight loss, decreased appetite and poor nutrition, and inactivity, often accompanied by dehydration, depressive symptoms, impaired immune function, and low cholesterol. Occurring in both acute and chronic forms, failure to thrive leads to impaired functional status, morbidity from infection, pressure sores, and, ultimately, increased mortality. Failure to thrive also leads to increases in institutionalization and health care costs. One example of promising research into this syndrome is the conduct of cross-cohort and longitudinal studies to determine the prevalence and the underlying risk factors precipitating failure to thrive. Another important example is the study of interventions to prevent or treat such consequences of failure to thrive as pressure sores and depression.

Impaired Postural Stability, Strength, and Mobility

This is a syndrome that includes the common problems of falls, dizziness, syncope, fractures, muscle weakness, and impaired mobility. These problems tend to occur increasingly in persons over the age of 75 and result in significant functional disability and dependence. Each year in the United States there are over 200,000 hip fractures—the majority of which are precipitated by falls—in persons over the age of 65 (Cummings et al., 1985). One specific research recommendation in this area is to determine the pathophysiologic mechanisms and other factors underlying recurrent falls and mobility impairment, including gait disorder and muscle atrophy. Further study is needed to explore effects of pharmacologic agents and other therapy (graded exercise) on improving or impairing some of these functions.

Mismanagement of Medications

The management of multiple medical conditions in older patients often involves several medications. Polypharmacy, defined as the taking of three or more medications on a regular basis, is found in a third of persons over the age of 65 (Nolan and O'Malley, 1988). Recent studies indicate that polypharmacy is a significant cause of morbidity and hospitalization among elderly patients (Williamson and Chopin, 1980; Ives et al., 1987; Grymonpre et al., 1988). Many of the geriatric syndromes described in this report occur as side effects of prescription medications. Yet, at the same time, many older persons' easily treated conditions are not managed aggressively enough with the appropriate pharmacologic agents.

This mismanagement of medications compromises independence and quality of life, and it increases the costs of health care. More studies of the fundamental pharmacodynamics of various medications in older individuals would forward clinical care in this area. Additionally, opportunity exists for excellent ground-breaking interdisciplinary investigation of medication use and effects that link basic clinical and behavioral science approaches. This might include gene delivery systems (cells carrying engineered genes), specific enzyme-blocking agents, and monoclonal antibodies.

Urinary Incontinence

Urinary incontinence, although it varies in intensity and in the degree to which its victims are disabled, is a highly prevalent, costly, morbid, and seriously neglected problem in elderly persons. The prevalence of urinary incontinence is approximately 30 percent in community-dwelling older persons (Diokno et al., 1986) and reaches 50 percent for those in nursing homes (Ouslander et al., 1982). Costs of incontinence are measured not only in terms of the financial burden of its management (e.g., linen changes; use of absorbent pads; and use of diapers, condoms, and catheters) and its clinical morbidity, but also in psychosocial terms. Our knowledge regarding the mechanisms underlying urinary incontinence and the appropriate approach to its control is rudimentary. There is a great need for clinical studies to determine the neuroanatomic and neurophysiologic basis of urinary incontinence and the efficacy and risk of treatment (e.g., drugs, surgery, training, and elimination of risk factors). Finally, there is an urgent need to develop new, effective, and safe treatments—preventive, ameliorative, or curative—for incontinence.

Delirium

Delirium, the development of acute confusional states, is a global disturbance of cognitive function accompanied by an alteration, and often fluctuation, in the level of attentiveness and, usually, consciousness. Delirium frequently is overlooked or misdiagnosed, and often mistaken for dementia. Approximately one-third of hospitalized elderly individuals develop an acute confusional state, markedly complicating their hospital course and dramatically increasing not only morbidity but also health care costs (Lipowski, 1989). Despite its high prevalence and tremendous morbidity and costs, little is known about the underlying mechanisms of or effective interventions for delirium.

- **The second research priority involves studies of the interaction of age-dependent physiological changes and important diseases in old age.**

The scientific and medical community needs to evaluate the interaction of age-related physiologic changes with diseases that either occur predominantly in aged populations or present different symptoms, course, or sequelae when occurring in the aged. This area of research is largely interdisciplinary since a number of lifestyle and socioenvironmental factors have an important influence on the emergence of disease in aging populations. Research on the interaction of aging and disease processes provides a critical link to issues of functional capacity since each major disease category mentioned in this report imposes a large burden on the aging population; prevention of or more effective intervention into these disorders might well reduce the onset of disability.

To effect the study of the interaction of aging in disease, research knowledge of biologic and physiologic processes from many levels must be integrated. Crucial to this effort is the appreciation that research gains in the areas of both normal and disease states act synergistically to increase our understanding of pathophysiologic mechanisms. This approach has been particularly well demonstrated in the use of molecular biological tools that delve into genetic regulatory processes that underlie the control of both normal and abnormal molecular and cellular processes. To gain an understanding of age-related pathophysiology, the medical and scientific community must exploit the most fundamental techniques of molecular and cell biology and apply them to the investigation of normal human aging. There is reason to be optimistic that a better-understood and better-mapped human genome, coupled with the application of now-standard techniques of reverse genetics, will allow the genetic contributions to many of these diseases to be defined specifically. This development, plus the extension to actual gene therapy of current techniques to introduce cells carrying engineered genes, may allow us to prevent, cure, or otherwise substantially modify many of these diseases.

Cardiovascular Disease

Cardiovascular disorders are a major target, for cardiac disease is the number one cause of death in persons over the age of 65 and cerebral vascular disease is the third most common cause of death in elderly persons (National Center for Health Statistics, 1989). Most of these disorders are due to atherosclerosis: excessive thickening and narrowing of coronary, cerebral, and peripheral arteries. Unfortunately, inadequate data address these problems because, to date, elderly persons have not been represented adequately in clinical studies of cardiovascular therapies. Thus, increased research on cardiovascular disorders among older persons is needed. Emphasis should be placed (1) on understanding the genetic as well as the environmental risk factors and the molecular basis of atherosclerosis, and (2) on developing standard and recombinant-based drug technologies as well as new approaches to prevent (in younger adults) and treat hypertension, lipid disorder, and the thrombotic complications of atherosclerosis. The role of nutrition, and the interaction of genetic and nutritional factors in the cause and prevention of these diseases, are important areas for future research.

Dementia, Pseudodementia, and Psychiatric Disorders

Recent studies have shown that dementia after age 75 reaches well over 40 percent; an overwhelming proportion of these patients have senile dementia of the Alzheimer's type (Hagnell et al., 1983; Sayetta, 1986). If dementia were cited on the death certificates of persons in whom it was a primary underlying disease, it would be the fourth or fifth leading cause of death in the United States (Weiler, 1987). Furthermore, in this country dementia now is the leading cause of institutionalization (Von Vostrand, 1979). Affective disorders are underreported in older persons even though they account for substantial disability in this age group (Finlayson and Martin, 1982). Although there are many outstanding research opportunities in this area, the greatest need is for studies linking basic and clinical approaches to the pathophysiology, cause, prevention, and treatment of Alzheimer's disease and other dementias. Excellent opportunities are available for basic molecular and cell biologic studies to determine the mechanisms and causes of central nervous system cell death in the aged, particularly the role of growth factors in central nervous system changes associated with both normal aging and injury. These studies should include assessment of cellular and molecular markers and new approaches to imaging and neurotransmitter mapping of the nervous system. Such studies clearly overlap with the research areas emphasized in Chapter 2. In addition, clinical studies that focus on management strategies for demented older persons have major interrelations with social, behavioral, and health services research agendas.

Musculoskeletal Disorders

Musculoskeletal disorders rank second to circulatory system diseases as a cause of both disability and health care costs in the United States. These conditions rank second in frequency as a reason for visits to physicians and third in frequency of hospitalization. Osteoarthritis is the most prevalent joint condition after age 65 (National Center for Health Statistics, 1989), and ranks second (after cardiovascular disease) in producing severe disability in those over age 60. Osteoporosis is also extremely common; annually, over one million osteoporosis-related fractures occur in the United States (Resnick and Greenspan, 1989). Fractures of the vertebral bodies and the hip are the two most common types of fracture in elderly persons, and both cause significant morbidity. Of those suffering from hip fracture, 50 percent never walk again (Melton and Riggs, 1983). Resultant costs from these disorders total more than $65 billion annually.

The application of restriction fragment-length polymorphism and other techniques of reverse genetics will help to provide the tools necessary to define the genetic basis of osteoarthritis and osteoporosis in many patients suffering from these common disorders. Such approaches should receive a high priority, particularly if current techniques of genetic engineering can be extended to gene replacement.

Infectious Disease and Immunosenescence

Infections, especially pneumonia and those of the urinary tract, are a major cause of disability and mortality in old persons. However, the exact extent of disability from infectious disorders in older people is largely unknown. Knowledge is incomplete about the prevention and treatment of infection in this population. Specific research opportunities include studies of the basic mechanisms of immune deficiency in older individuals, including changes at the cellular level involving T-cell subsets, natural killer cells, macrophages, and receptor-mediated responses. Vaccine development needs to take into account the special characteristics of the elderly population. Vaccines that can bypass the need for immune T cells and vaccines made with live attenuated organisms with antigen attached to a rigid backbone may be more effective in old people. These efforts should utilize new technologies such as DNA recombinant vaccines and genetically engineered attenuated viruses. The focus on immunosenescence is also directly related to the next research focus, cancer in older persons, since impaired immunity contributes to cancer development.

Neoplasia

Cancer and its related complications are the number two cause of death in persons over the age of 65 (National Center for Health Statistics, 1989); for elderly persons death due to cancer is the second leading cause of lost years of life. The basis for the age-associated frequency of and disability related to cancer is unknown. In addition, efforts at primary (e.g., prevent onset of disease), secondary (e.g., prevent onset of complications of disease), and tertiary (e.g., treat complications of disease) prevention of cancer have been limited almost entirely to the younger population. For example, little information exists on the efficacy of smoking cessation programs and the efficacy and toxicity of standard chemotherapeutic regimens for those 65 years or older. As with several of the other suggested areas of research identified in this report, there is a clear and substantial overlap between the clinical research related to neoplasia and the focus on aging and cell proliferation suggested in the basic biomedical component of this research agenda. Reverse genetics, recombinant DNA products, and delivery systems using gene transfer approaches should be particularly valuable in this area. Interactions between environmental (e.g., carcinogens and nutritional factors) and genetic factors in the cause and prevention of cancer warrant intensive study.

Disorders of Metabolism and Homeostasis

Strong epidemiologic evidence indicates that metabolic dysfunctions have significant impact on the pathogenesis of numerous disorders affecting the health of older individuals. Metabolic problems may precede the development of clinical manifestations of disease, accelerating the progression of atherosclerosis, hypertension, neuropathy, and musculoskeletal disease. Disorders of metabolism and homeostasis influence the onset and severity of most of the alterations described elsewhere in this report. The metabolic disorders considered in generating these recommendations include diabetes mellitus, altered muscle metabolism, altered bone mineral metabolism, and lipid disorders. Intensive studies should be undertaken to clarify the pathophysiology and genetic basis and to elucidate the long-term complications of these disorders in elderly individuals. Research on relationships among genetic, pathogenic, and nutritional factors will be of great value.

ADDITIONAL RESEARCH OPPORTUNITIES

Although the committee emphasizes the foregoing areas of research for priority consideration, other areas should not be neglected in the research agenda on aging. These additional opportunities include dental and oral problems in aging, especially the prevention and treatment of periodontal disease, cancer of the mouth, and orofacial pain; diagnosis and treatment of neurogenic dysphagia; investigation of hearing impairment, its prevention, and its treatment; study of conditions (particularly glaucoma, cataracts, and macular degeneration) contributing to loss of vision in the aged; and various skin conditions associated with aging (keratomas, skin cancer, and dry skin).

While each of the foregoing research areas leads to detailed specific secondary research objectives, each area also represents the interface of several disciplines. Major opportunities in clinical geriatric research exist in interfaces between physician-scientists and colleagues from the social and behavioral sciences. Increasingly, productive interaction between basic and clinical scientists is resulting in research strategies and protocols that provide the opportunity for application of molecular biological and other basic science techniques to clinical problems and populations.

RESOURCE RECOMMENDATIONS

The ambitious, though appropriate and overdue, clinical research program recommended in this chapter can only be implemented effectively if two major resources become available. The first is funding to support the specific research projects that flow from the two major thematic areas in this chapter (described in greater detail in the Executive Summary and Recommendations for Funding). Additional funding is required to launch an effective research program in the major consensus areas identified as most deserving of support. There would be little delay in the development of excellent research proposals in these areas since the National Institute on Aging (NIA) and other federal agencies already have a substantial number of approved but unfunded research proposals with excellent priority scores. The additional research funds could be applied to such applications, thus raising the level of support from the current less than one in four (24 percent) to one in two.

However, allocation of substantial funds to support research projects will not ensure the successful completion of the clinical research agenda. The second major necessary resource is professional talent. For example, a recent IOM report (IOM, 1987; Rowe et al., 1987) shows a critical need for the development of scientists with a commitment to and appropriate training for research in geriatrics. Both basic biomedical and more clinically oriented investigators are desperately needed in all disciplines related to clinical research in older persons. Two strategies are suggested to attract young health professionals and Ph.D. students into the fields of geriatrics and gerontology. First, increased funds are needed to establish the ongoing fellowship and postdoctoral programs that will be the lifeblood of the next generation of clinical gerontologists. These funds would permit graduation of an additional 200 fellows and postdoctoral students per year, as well as provide support for 180 junior faculty and midlevel investigators who have recently moved into the fields of geriatrics and gerontology.

A second strategy to develop a cadre of outstanding clinically oriented investigators in geriatrics and gerontology is the addition of at least 10 highly sophisticated Geriatric Research and Training Centers (Claude Pepper Centers) to the current three supported by the NIA. This strategy has been recommended in a separate report of the IOM that focuses on workforce needs in geriatrics. Subsequent to that report, enabling legislation has been drafted and adopted by Congress. These centers would be developed in the setting of currently well-established academic research and clinical programs on aging. A moderate amount of core support should be provided to these centers for continuity of key research personnel and ongoing efforts; however, such centers would be expected to compete for additional research funds on a continuing basis to ensure that their work remains current and is peer reviewed. The primary goal of these centers would be to produce substantial numbers of very well-trained, clinical-research-oriented investigators. To date, three centers have been funded. Ample expertise already exists at enough academic programs to warrant immediate funding of 10 additional centers, followed by funding of further centers over the next several years as the need is demonstrated.

Finally, it is abundantly clear that the facilities and infrastructure available in the United States to support the research enterprise are seriously deficient. Accordingly, the committee recommends additional support for infrastructure and for construction of new research space and renovation of outdated space.

CROSSCUTTING ISSUES

Clinical research in geriatrics and gerontology requires an approach that engages many disciplines. Insights from molecular and cell biology provide a basic biomedical foundation for much clinical investigation, including newer therapies for Alzheimer's disease and the diagnosis of age-associated cancers such as carcinoma of the colon. Behavioral and social research and the insights offered by studies in health care delivery make possible clinical programs to study the responses of older people to illness, and to find better ways of intervening to reduce disability and morbidity among the aged.

Of equal importance in clinical research are crosscutting issues that involve gender differences in response to illness or in the metabolic disposition of drugs as well as racial and ethnic variation in the way older individuals experience illness, both from a patient care perspective and from the vantage of exploring differences in physiological response to disease. An example of the influence of gender differences on outcome of disease is seen in the lower rates of morbidity and mortality in women who have hypertension than in men with hypertension. Racial differences also appear to influence prognosis in some diseases; higher death and complication rates occur in hypertensive black men than in white men.

Another critical crosscutting issue is that of ethics in clinical research. Obtaining informed consent from cognitively impaired elders, using drugs with high risk to benefit ratios in geriatric populations, and resolving conflicts arising from confrontations between medical paternalism and the need for patient autonomy are all examples of the pervasiveness of this issue in clinical geriatric medicine and in geriatric and gerontological research.

REFERENCES

Branch, L. G., S. Katz, K. Kniedmann, and J. A. Papsidero. 1984. A prospective study of functional status among community elders. American Journal of Public Health 74:266-268.

Cummings, S. R., J. L. Kelsey, M. C. Nevitt, and K. J. O'Dowd. 1985. Epidemiology of osteoporosis and osteoporotic fractures. Epidemiology Review 7:178-208.

Dawson, D., G. Hendershop, and J. Fulton. 1987. Aging in the Eighties: Functional Limitations of Individuals 65 and Over. Advance Data No. 133, National Center for Health Statistics. Washington, D.C.: U.S. Government Printing Office.

Diokno, A. C., B. M. Brock, M. B. Brown, and A. R. Herzog. 1986. Prevalence of urinary incontinence and other urological symptoms in the non-institutionalized elderly. Journal of Urology 136:1022-1025.

Finlayson, R. E. and L. M. Martin. 1982. Recognition and management of depression in the elderly. Mayo Clinic Proceedings 57:115-120.

Grymonpre, R. E., P. A. Mitenko, D. S. Sitar, F. Y. Aoke, and P. R. Montgomery. 1988. Drug-associated hospital admissions in older medical patients. Journal of the American Geriatrics Society 36:1094-1098.

Hagnell, O., J. Lanke, B. Rorsman, R. Ohman, and L. Ojesjö. 1983. Current trends in the incidence of senile and multi-infarct dementia. Archives of Psychiatry and Neurological Science 233:423-428.

Institute of Medicine. 1987. Academic geriatrics for the year 2000. Report of the Committee on Leadership for Academic Geriatric Medicine. Journal of the American Geriatrics Society 35:773-791.

Institute of Medicine. 1989. Effectiveness Initiative: Setting Priorities for Clinical Conditions. Washington, D.C.: National Academy Press.

Institute of Medicine. 1990a. Effectiveness and Outcomes in Health Care. Washington, D.C.: National Academy Press.

Institute of Medicine. 1990b. The Second 50 Years: Promoting Health and Preventing Disability. Washington, D.C.: National Academy Press.

Ives, T. J., E. J. Bentz, and R. E. Gwyther. 1987. Drug-related admissions to a family medicine inpatient service. Archives of Internal Medicine 147:1117-1120.

Lipowski, Z. J. 1989. Delirium in the elderly patient. New England Journal of Medicine 320:578-582.

Melton, L. J., III and B. L. Riggs. 1983. The epidemiology of age-related fractures. In The Osteoporotic Syndrome, L. V. Avioli, ed. New York: Grune and Stratton.

National Center for Health Statistics. 1985. National Health Interview Survey. Vital and Health Statistics, Series 10, No. 150. DHHS Pub. No. (PHS) 85-1578. Washington, D.C.: U.S. Government Printing Office.

National Center for Health Statistics. 1989. Vital and Health Statistics Report,

No. 173 and 37, No. 5, Supplement. Washington, D.C.: U.S. Government Printing Office.

Nolan, L. and K. O'Malley. 1988. Prescribing for the elderly. Part 20. Prescribing patterns: Differences due to age. Journal of the American Geriatrics Society 36:245-254.

Ouslander, J. G., R. L. Kane, and I. B. Abrass. 1982. Urinary incontinence in elderly nursing home patients. Journal of the American Medical Association 248:1194-1198.

Resnick, N., and S. L. Greenspan. 1989. Senile osteoporosis reconsidered. Journal of the American Medical Association 261:1025-1029.

Rowe, J. W., E. Grossman, and E. Bond. 1987. Academic geriatrics for the year 2000: An Institute of Medicine report. New England Journal of Medicine 316:1425-1428.

Sayetta, R. B. 1986. Rates of senile dementia-Alzheimer's type in the Baltimore longitudinal study. Journal of Chronic Disease 39:271-285.

Von Vostrand, J. 1979. The National Nursing Home Survey: 1977 Summary for the United States, National Center for Health Statistics. Vital and Health Statistics, Series 13, No. 43. DHEW Pub. No. 43 (PHS) 79-1794. Washington, D.C.: U.S. Government Printing Office.

Weiler, P. 1987. The public health impact of Alzheimer's disease. American Journal of Public Health 77:1157-1158.

Williams, T. F. 1988. Rehabilitation: Goals and Approaches in Older People. Pp. 136-143 in Geriatric Medicine, 2nd Ed., J. W. Rowe and R. W. Besdine, eds. Boston: Little, Brown.

Williamson, J., and J. Chopin. 1980. Adverse reactions to prescribed drugs in the elderly: A multicenter investigation. Age and Ageing 9:73-80.

4

Behavioral and Social Sciences

Recent behavioral and social research has advanced our understanding of the aging process, the health and well-being of older adults, and the experience of growing older in our society. Three conclusions emerge from a review of this research: (1) sociocultural contexts are an important influence on aging processes; (2) significant variability in aging exists among individuals and between social groups; and (3) skills, behavior, and competence can be modified in old age. Increased length of life, which has dramatically altered the age structure of populations, coupled with changes in social policy and family structure, underscores the need to know more about the nature of aging today and its likely effects on future generations.

The primary goal of research in health and aging must be to compress and diminish the duration of morbidity, disability, and suffering during the extra years provided by increased life expectancy and to enhance both productivity and the quality of life during that time. Because of the complexity of life processes, a considerable portion of this research must be multidisciplinary, longitudinal, and cohort sequential, working within existing knowledge, methodology, and resources. For example, behavioral and social studies can contribute to the understanding of the response to clinical interventions or can make clear the factors that influence older persons' access to and participation in health care services. Although the traditional approach to research is featured in this review, long-term payoffs from less-established but promising areas of research should not be neglected.

The significance of research discoveries in behavioral and social research on aging can be interpreted in light of three important themes, developed in the next section, bearing on how individuals age, experience aging, and respond to aging: (1) the dynamic interaction of older individuals and sociocultural contexts, (2) differentiation among older individuals and in the aging process itself, and (3) modifiability through interventions to improve the quality of aging.

Approaches to the scientific study of sociological and behavioral factors in aging include (1) refinement of measurement and analytic instruments, (2) cooperation and coordination by different disciplines in large-scale investigations using carefully selected, culturally representative panels to be followed longitudinally and cohort sequentially, and (3) application and evaluation of research findings through systematic field studies to test the appropriateness of particular intervention techniques.

JUSTIFICATION AND MAJOR THEMES

Fundamental advances in the study of aging have resulted from the demonstration that factors in the social and physical environment extrinsic to the individual can dramatically alter the course of aging. Thus, the process of aging is highly mutable and susceptible to interventions of a social and behavioral nature. The committee believes that social and behavioral interventions derived from the research agenda described below will materially improve the functioning and quality of life of older persons.

Research also emphasizes the fact that, because aging is a lifelong process, it is useful to study both the multiple determinants of successful aging and the causes and consequences of dysfunction and disability. Finally, research has demonstrated the importance of embedding the study of aging in the broader sociocultural context: race, ethnicity, gender, cultural identity, and the social environment.

The Dynamic Interaction of Individuals and Sociocultural Contexts

Genetic and other biological forces affect individual health and behavior within specific sociocultural contexts. The effects and mechanisms of these interactions affecting psychosocial aspects of health and aging need to be understood. At least four bodies of research highlight these complex dynamics. These include studies of (1) comparative aging in different societies, cultures, racial/ethnic groups, and other subpopulations; (2) the influences on aging of different environments (including geographic, workplace, and treatment environments), living arrangements, and other forms of material and social support; (3) the effects on behavioral and health outcomes of older persons' individual characteristics coupled with the varying opportunities and constraints of different social milieus; and (4) the brain/behavior relationship.

Medical research can no longer be separated artificially from sociological, economic, or psychological research. The social contexts in which individuals develop and age influence the length of their lives, their health, their ability to make decisions or cope with the demands of their conditions, their functional capacities, and the way they feel. Indeed, each of these factors influences the others. The natural laboratory provided by differences among subpopulations and subcultures in our own society, between our society and others, and between those who grew up at one time in history and those who grew up at another evidences the fact that growing up and growing old varies, for example, if one is a member of a developing society; if one is black, female, or poor; or if one is of a particular birth cohort.

Contemporary social and behavioral research in aging displays an increasingly sophisticated view of the dynamic effects of culture, social setting, and context on individual behavior (Featherman and Lerner, 1985; Maddox, and Campbell, 1985; Campbell and O'Rand, 1988; Riley, 1988; Spenner, 1988). One example of such research (Moos, 1974, 1980) illustrates efforts to measure and examine the varied settings in terms of environmental and individual characteristics and the interactions between the two. Several important conclusions have been suggested. First, the characteristics of the setting—whether structural or interpersonal factors—affect outcome. Second, personal characteristics, such as the individual capacity for cognitive appraisal and coping can, to a degree, compensate for repressive controlling environments. Third, the "fit" between personal characteristics and independence-enhancing environments predicts a beneficial health outcome. Last, the social processes that route individuals toward beneficial milieus are as important as providing a beneficial environment in the first instance.

Differentiation

Both within and across societies, the older population is extremely heterogeneous; moreover, aging has varied substantially over historical time. People arrive at the end of life by different routes, and societies influence these routes in varied but consequential ways. Social and psychological factors affect both how individuals and the broader society age and experience aging. This variability is the best evidence for modifiability in later life. Aging is dependent on gender and ethnic, economic, political, and educational circumstances. Lifestyle, risks of illness and dependency, and functional ability also affect how one ages. Research by sociologists, economists, historians, and anthropologists has documented why references to "elderly persons," the "minority elderly persons," or "the older woman" are necessarily inaccurate and misleading (Clark and Spengler, 1980; Keith, 1985; Verbrugge, 1985; Maddox, 1987b).

Although observed variation in aging surely has a biological component, the list of explanatory factors must include those that are predominantly social and behavioral. Research has demonstrated that sanitation, food, and clean water, as well as adequate income, education, and housing, have powerful effects on life expectancy, health, and functioning. In the most impoverished developing countries, for example, average life expectancy is about half of that in developed societies (Torrey et al., 1987). To be poor or black in the United States costs an individual, on average, 5 or 6 years of life expectancy. Poor people, who typically are also undereducated, tend to be underinsured, to use health care facilities less effectively, and to be less likely to adopt healthful lifestyles (Berkman, 1988).

In our society the differential allocation of resources—jobs or related income—by gender or ethnicity increases the risk of poverty, illness, and premature death in later life. Chronological age is only a crude predictor of behavior or health. Although the risk of functional impairment increases with age (Manton, 1988), people in their 80s have a 50 percent chance of continuing sufficiently free of disability, so as to be capable of self-care (Katz et al., 1983), although this figure decreases as one approaches the late 80s. Older individuals differ in their sense of self-control (Rodin et al., 1985; Rodin, 1986), in their capacity to cope with illness or other life challenges (Siegler and Costa, 1985), and in their risk of mental disability (Blazer and Meador, 1988; George, 1989). Such differences are dependent on social, behavioral, psychological, lifestyle, and cohort characteristics.

Modifiability

From this knowledge of differential approaches to old age stems the concept of the modifiability of aging. Improvements in socioeconomic circumstances can simultaneously improve health and well-being in the young and old. Recent research shows that many aspects of the course and outcome of the aging process are plastic—that is, open to intervention. For example, investigators have developed ways in which to restore and enhance learning and memory apparently lost in very old individuals (Schaie and Willis, 1986) and to enhance self-esteem, thus enabling previously passive, institutionalized elders to take better care of themselves (Rodin et al., 1985, 1990). Because studies documenting the potential modifiability of aging have tended to focus on reducing age-related decrements in the health of individuals, research is needed to define more broadly the areas and limits of the modifiability of aging, particularly in terms of enhancing existing skills and learning in later life.

RESEARCH PRIORITIES

Three major research priorities flow from these themes.

- **The first priority is investigation of the basic social and psychological processes of aging and the specific mechanisms underlying the interrelationships among social, psychological, behavioral, and biological aging functions.**
- **The second priority is research that addresses issues of population dynamics, including the question of whether morbidity is being postponed commensurate with increases in longevity.**
- **The third priority is research that examines how social structures and changes in those structures affect aging.**

These priorities should be seen as the cognitive precursors to specific research questions that will examine issues related to health and functioning—the primary focus of this report. In formulating the research priorities, and in discussing the priorities listed below, the committee has not examined needed research addressing the full array of societal and specific behavioral issues and questions posed by an aging society, such as economic and political implications. The latter, however, represent an equally crucial research agenda.

- **Investigation of the basic social and psychological processes of aging and the specific mechanisms underlying the interrelationships among social, psychological, behavioral, and biological aging functions should be undertaken.**

A search for the mechanisms of the interrelationships among hitherto separate disciplines would include studies of (1) the social, psychological, and behavioral variables that predict health, longevity, functional ability, and well-being in individuals and (2) the most effective techniques for maintaining and improving general physical and mental health, and functioning. Once such mechanisms are identified, different intervention models need to be compared.

Biologists have emphasized the inevitability and unidirectionality of decline (Rockstein and Sussman, 1979; Finch and Schneider, 1985). Psychologists, however, have found that some behavioral capacities are multidirectional: some improve over the life course, some remain stable, and others decline (Woodruff-Pak, 1988). Further, because individuals are adaptive in their behavioral adjustment to biological decline in aging, behavioral decline often is minimal. Moreover, understanding the range of limits of physiological decline and its consequence for behavior is an important priority for future research.

One of the most exciting frontiers involves the examination of the interaction among behavior, central nervous system structure and function, and neuroendocrines and other hormonal factors. Examples include investigation of the relationship between memory function and such central nervous system structures as the hippocampus and cerebellum (Berger et al., 1986) and research on stress-related environmental, psychological, and hormonal factors that lead to anatomic changes in the brain (see cerebral atrophy under extreme stress: Jensen et al., 1982; Finch, 1987). Although extensive descriptive literature exists on both physiological and psychological changes in advancing age, only limited information is available on specific behavioral correlates of specific biological changes. Data on specific interactions between biological and psychosocial factors are even more sparse. It is suspected, for example, that adverse changes in the synchrony between the autonomic and central nervous systems in advancing age may affect intellectual performance, particularly in jobs or tasks requiring complex decision making.

Despite the recognition that the major health problems of older people are chronic, little attention has been paid to behavioral and social interventions to reduce excessive disability and provide new treatment and management strategies. Some key issues for researchers include rehabilitative strategies to maintain or restore function, treatment of the social or emotional barriers to rehabilitation, and compliance with medical regimens. A variety of behavioral interventions—biofeedback in hypertension, for example—appear promising (Zarit, in press). Behavioral interventions also can be used to enhance performance of older people (Rodin, 1986).

The movement from work to retirement is one of the most important life-course decisions facing middle-aged and older workers. It has significant public policy implications, deriving from federal regulations, personnel policies, and decisions of workers. New social and economic surveys need to link business characteristics, such as pension plans and retiree health insurance, with individual career and retirement decisions. It is important to examine the age-productivity relationship in different settings (IOM, 1981; Sterns and Alexander, 1987; Spenner, 1988) so as to identify matches and mismatches between productive capacity of older workers and the personnel preferences and policies of business firms.

Adopting a life-course perspective that views today's younger adults as tomorrow's older adults should be paired with monitoring social change and the changing sociodemographic and health characteristics of populations. To the extent that children and younger adults at risk can be identified and helped, the elder population of the future will enjoy better health and well-being.

Research should be designed to provide a clearer understanding of individual differences in sensory, cognitive, and behavioral aging, particularly as these differences reflect relationships between brain and behavior, environment and behavior, and society and behavior. Applied and clinical research can translate into practice what is known about the modifiability of risk factors, skills, learning, and memory. Evaluation procedures need to be improved and effective interventions devised.

- **Research that addresses issues of population dynamics, including the question of whether morbidity is being postponed commensurate with increases in longevity, is a further high priority.**

Descriptive demography and epidemiology and techniques of population estimation have improved substantially in recent years (Hogan, 1985; Myers, 1985; Torrey et al., 1987; Guilford, 1988). Apart from the significance of immigration, two high priorities for research include (1) improved and continued forecasts of the future number of older persons, both in developed and developing nations, and (2) estimates of the proportion of those people who will be able or unable to function independently. Important work on forecasting is now under way in several research sites and is in continuing need of support. For the United States, sophisticated forecasts are now suggesting that, given a degree of control over well-known risk factors for heart disease, the size of the older population in the twenty-first century would exceed even the current high estimates (Manton, 1988). Unquestionably, the society will be confronted with unprecedented numbers of both healthy and disabled older people, and it is of critical importance that more be known about the interaction of factors—behavioral, social, and biological—that influence the time of onset of morbidity and disability as life expectancy continues to increase.

Comparative studies, such as epidemiological studies of cardiovascular disease among Japanese in different locations, are suggested as timely and useful in helping us to understand the dynamics of adaptive life transitions in varied groups. Identifying factors that enhance active life expectancy of ethnic minorities is an essential step in developing effective policy to assist minority elderly persons. Research on population dynamics needs to give special attention to at-risk populations—in particular, those subpopulations at high risk for poverty, social isolation, underemployment, inadequate education, illness, and inaccessibility to health care. Higher-priority attention should be given to such subpopulations as the poor, women, and minorities.

The physical and mental health of men and women in the United States differ in significant but paradoxical ways. Women have a higher incidence of transitory illness and a higher prevalence of nonfatal chronic diseases, they report more symptoms of illness, and they are major consumers of health care services. Women under age 65 experience more injuries, bed disability, and restricted activity days than men; this gender difference becomes even more pronounced at age 65 (Minkler and Stone, 1983). Maddox (1987a) found that women were more likely to be impaired and to be impaired earlier than men; when socioeconomic status was equalized, however, this difference disappeared. Yet, on average, women live 8 years longer than men (Verbrugge, 1985, 1988). These differences provide an obvious opportunity for cohort-sequential longitudinal research to document whether observed gender differences in morbidity and well-being are persisting or changing over time.

It is important that research also strives to identify and explain psychological variables both as predictors of health, longevity, and functional disability and as ends in themselves. Psychological and behavioral variables may not only contribute to biological aging, but may also be the behavioral representation of physiological dysfunction. In addition, certain psychological states need to be identified as conditions that must be managed in the aging process. Equally, this research necessitates detailed analyses of existing databases and the creation of new databases that contain information on health histories and psychological functioning to allow testing of the reciprocal effects of illness, lifestyles, personality variables, and psychological competence.

- **Research should be undertaken to study the manner in which social structures and changes in those structures affect aging.**

Just as individuals change, so too do social structures; observations of old age today show neither what old age was like in the past nor what it will be like in the future (Bengtson et al., 1985; Riley et al., 1987; Riley, 1988). It is necessary to identify stability and change in social structures and to show how stability or change affects the performance, productivity, health, and well-being of older adults. Special attention should be paid to such traditional subpopulations as ethnic and racial minorities and older women for whom social status and change entail increased risk to health. Although family structure and function continue to change, research points to a continuation of intergenerational contact and support, even when families are separated geographically (Sussman, 1985). Kinship ties still bond generations (Bengtson et al., 1985), and families continue to be the dominant source of social support in all societies (Horowitz, 1985; Hagestad, 1987).

Because of the social changes experienced in recent decades in the United States, further research is required on stability and change in living arrangements and exchange relationships. The changing structure of families and the implications of these changes for social support and caregiving demand special attention (Oppenheimer, 1982). The work force, the labor market, and the family responsibilities of women, for example, have been characterized by considerable change, but the effects of these changes have not been monitored adequately in research. The knowledge that family and labor force composition have changed does not give us the needed evidence for sound estimates of how these changes will affect the availability of social support for dependent older persons in the future. There has been little study, for example, of the implications of four-generation families, the conditions under which outside support services may affect informal family care, or how family support can be supplemented effectively by community services.

In the past decade sociologists, psychologists, and economists have looked at the relationships among work, retirement, and productivity. As our nation confronts a critical shortage of workers, increasing numbers of able older persons are spending two to three decades of their lives in retirement. Research is needed to specify what changes in social structure could provide productive opportunities for these older people and to examine how current trends in work, retirement, and productivity are experienced by aging individuals; how they affect physical and psychosocial functioning; and how they may result in loss of productivity. Studies that contribute to the better understanding and design of assessment techniques for evaluating work capacity and prolonging work careers of older adults clearly are needed. Additional studies are needed as well to understand the effects of the policies and decisions of business leadership on the hiring and retirement of older workers, and behavioral research is needed to discover the mechanisms that link changes in social structures (education, job experience, income patterns, and family constellations) to individual differences in maintenance of psychological competence, well-being, and adaptive capacity as people age (Schooler and Schaie, 1987; Schaie and Schooler, 1989).

Whereas the dynamics of poverty among adults are increasingly understood (Duncan, 1984), fewer data are available about the dynamics of moving into and out of poverty. Lifetime earnings, personal savings, and pension coverage provide the resources for retirement, but income and wealth can be depleted during retirement by the death of a spouse, health crises, and/or adverse financial events (Burkhauser et al., 1988). The economic status of older people has been little studied; more research on this subject is needed to untangle the complex interrelationships among aging, economics, gender, racial/ethnic status, and health as measured by mortality, disability, chronic illness, and institutionalization.

Contextual variables are known to exert significant influence on behavior and performance. The mechanisms through which specific changes, events, or length of exposure to certain milieus influence behavioral outcome, such as role performance, health, and sense of well-being, are less clear. They must be addressed from a variety of perspectives, and caution is indicated in extrapolating from one cohort to another, particularly concerning expectations, attitudes, and preferences among older people. How social structure may affect psychological and biological aging may be explicated as well by study of the impact of social factors upon control processes that influence an individual's sense of effectiveness over the life course (Rodin et al., 1985; Rodin et al., in press).

ADDITIONAL RESEARCH OPPORTUNITIES

These include the following:

• Social research: (1) Study the characteristics of employment, workplaces, and older individuals who are associated with continued productive activity in lifelong jobs or in new careers; (2) study how actual performance and expectations about performance of older people are affected by changing technology and examine the efforts of firms to use training and job respecification to make technological changes as age neutral as possible; and (3) develop and apply a multidimensional quality of life index to identify contributing fac-

tors among subpopulations for whom the index is low (e.g., the very old or minorities).
• Behavioral research: (1) Study the psychological concomitants of illness and how these affect self-care and response to formal care; (2) study the comparative effectiveness of different modalities in the treatment of chronic mental disorders; and (3) examine the effect of behavioral and social intervention on the outcome of long-term illness.

METHODOLOGICAL NEEDS

The committee suggests that three methodological approaches be used to carry out the new research agenda in behavioral and social investigation. These are as follows: (1) refined measurement and analytic instruments such as tests, scales, and models for forecasting or analysis; (2) cooperative multidisciplinary large-scale investigations utilizing multicultural, diverse populations studied over time and cohort sequentially; and (3) studies of intervention techniques utilizing the findings of the foregoing research.

Tests and Instruments

Examples of new and improved measurements include (1) measures of functioning that build on current activities of living scales; (2) psychological and other behavioral assessment techniques that are age fair and culturally fair, such as tests of skills, abilities, knowledge, and capacities appropriate for older people and people in different population subgroups; (3) measures of social contexts such as home, workplace, and community; (4) more accurate ways to measure behavioral and social components of illnesses such as Alzheimer's disease; (5) improved techniques for longitudinal and cohort analysis; and (6) modeling techniques to facilitate trend prediction.

Coordination of Large-Scale Research

Although multidisciplinary research is difficult and costly, it is the only way to address many of the central issues of interrelationships and interactions among the variables and processes discussed above. These issues include demographic and epidemiological matters related to the postponement of morbidity, antecedents and consequences of health differences and sequencing among different groups, dimensions of caregiving (including effectiveness, duration, and outcome), effects of different strategies on financing long-term care, and the relation between age productivity and retirement, among others.

Field Intervention Studies

Large-scale behavioral field trials are needed to test hypotheses and evaluate recommendations for interventions based on the findings from the studies described above. These need to be systematic and of sufficient duration to observe long-term consequences and should include strategies to maintain and improve such health and cognitive functions as memory, new learning, and adaptations, as well as designs for home and workplace that would allow older people to maintain and prolong productivity and independent living.

Although large-scale longitudinal research projects are necessary to implement the research agenda, the importance of small-sample studies to enhance in-depth understanding about the processes of aging must not be ignored. These studies are less costly to implement, often provide information on a relatively short-term basis, and can, for example, gather data on individual performance that are "averaged out" in larger studies.

RESOURCE RECOMMENDATIONS

Significant additional resources will be necessary to undertake the needed behavioral and social science research agenda in aging in the major priority areas. The funds to acquire these resources are described in detail in the Executive Summary and Recommendations for Funding. Despite large growth in the federal commitment to health research in the past decades, the social and behavioral sciences actually have lost ground relative to other areas of research—a trend that must be stopped if the potential of this research agenda is to be realized.

Supports for behavioral and social research on aging in 1989 were estimated at $80–$100 million from the federal government and $10–$15 million from nonfederal sources such as foundations (Behavioral and Social Research Program, NIA). Based on the calculation of the dollars committed to behavioral and social research on aging, an estimate of the capacity for high-quality research, and the additional monies necessary to develop the new initiatives identified here, the total budget for age-related behavioral and social research should be increased by more than 100 percent over current expenditures, with the additional funds to be phased in over a 5-year period. The recommended distribution of additional funds for the research initiatives should support studies of social, psychological, behavioral, and biological interrelationships; "at-risk" populations; population dynamics; and changing social structures.

These resources involve (1) increasing the funding rate of NIA and other NIH approved research program grants (RPGs) on aging from one in four (24 percent) to one in two; (2) providing training for an additional 200 investigators per year in behavioral and social science; and (3) a one-time cost for construction. New resources will include a share in ten multidisciplinary research and training centers added to the current three centers (Claude Pepper Centers) supported by the NIA and participation in an expanded scientific infrastructure (laboratories, computer support, long-range population studies, and increased linkage to such existing databases as the Health Care Financing Administration Medicare data tapes).

The increasing isolation of older persons (one-third live alone), the burden of psychologically disabled older persons on families, and the presence of serious affective disorders (older white males have the highest suicide rate) among elderly persons point up the urgent need for research that leads to better management of social and behavioral problems in the older population.

CROSS-DISCIPLINARY AND CROSSCUTTING ISSUES

Basic biomedical and clinical researchers have only recently begun to examine the influence of gender, race, culture, ethnicity, and social class on biological processes and clinical presentations. These and other social and behavioral issues cut across the disciplines and offer opportunities for further investigation and understanding in the field of aging.

Gender

The difference in life expectancy at birth between the sexes was small for those born in 1900, but it has widened considerably over the century. Much of this difference can be ascribed to changes in child-bearing practice and other lifestyle factors as well as to tobacco-related deaths and heart disease. Social and behavioral gender differences in morbidity, particularly as related to chronic conditions, suggest many promising research areas, such as the gender-specific response to social isolation and psychological disorders; differences in the relation of social supports to functional status; the differential effects of gender in pension income, social role expectations, labor force participation, and responsibilities for caregiving; interactions among neuroendocrine and other hormones; and cognitive and psychological status. Potentially significant are the many connections of this research with work in clinical science and health services delivery research as it relates to alterability of risk factors, appropriateness and effectiveness of interventions, utilization, service delivery, and many other areas.

Race and Ethnicity, Socioeconomic Status, and Other Cultural Factors

As is the case with gender, the cultural factors associated with race and ethnicity present important variables across and among the disciplines of aging. For example, racial and ethnic differences in metabolizing certain drugs and substances are confounded by cultural variables in the use of these substances, definition and presentation of symptoms, other illness behaviors, and acceptance of treatment regimens. In addition, an understanding of the effects of racial and ethnic-cultural differences in resource allocation is critical in explaining clinical, social, and psychological differences in aging and in health care service utilization. Moreover, race and ethnicity may well be contributing factors to underlying basic biological processes or their manifestations in old age.

Population Dynamics

Issues of population dynamics include accurate estimation and prediction of population trends in longevity, mortality, morbidity, and functional status. These dynamics also have major linkages with health services delivery concerns about access, availability of services, financing, system design, and policy formation. However, these issues, particularly as they concern estimates of the health and functional problems most likely to face large numbers of elderly people in the coming decades, also have connections to basic biomedical and clinical research in terms of predicting problems and defining important areas of research.

Brain, Environment, Society, and Behavior

Some of the age-related deficits in memory performance and cognitive function are amenable to understanding at the neurobiological level. But the question of the extent of memory deficit due to deterioration of basic storage mechanisms in the brain in contrast to those due to altered modulatory processes also requires a better understanding of the related psychological and psychosocial processes. Moreover, the interaction of the brain with aspects of the environment—physiological, physical, and social—is also poorly understood (Finch, 1987). For example, environmental stress can influence sleep patterns, which can then reflect on brain activity and the mental and emotional sequelae. Such interactions demand both crosscutting and cross-disciplinary approaches to further our essential knowledge and understanding.

REFERENCES

Bengtson, V., N. Cutler, D. Mangen, and V. Marshall. 1985. Generations, cohorts and relations between age groups. Pp. 304-338 in Handbook of Aging and the Social Sciences, R. Binstock and E. Shanas, eds. New York: Van Nostrand Reinhold.

Berger, T. W., S. D. Berry, and R. F. Thompson. 1986. Role of the hippocampus in classical conditioning of aversive and appetitive behaviors. Pp. 203-239 in The Hippocampus, vol. 4, R. L. Isaacson and K. H. Pribam, eds. New York: Plenum.

Berkman, L. 1988. The changing and heterogeneous nature of aging and longevity: A social and biomedical perspective. Pp. 37-70 in Varieties of Aging: Annual Review of Gerontology and Geriatrics, vol. 8, G. Maddox and P. Lawton, eds. New York: Springer Publishing.

Blazer, D., and K. Meador. 1988. The social psychiatry of later life. Pp. 283-294 in Handbook of Social Psychiatry, A. Henderson and D. Burrows, eds. New York: Elsevier.

Burkhauser, R., K. Holden, and D. Feaster. 1988. Incidence, timing and events associated with poverty: A dynamic view on poverty in retirement. Journal of Gerontology 43:546-552.

Campbell, R. T., and A. O'Rand. 1988. Settings and sequence: The heuristics of aging research. Pp. 58-82 in Emergent Theories of Aging, J. Birren and V. Bengtson, eds. New York: Springer Publishing.

Clark, R., and J. Spengler. 1980. The Economics of Individual and Population Aging. New York: Cambridge University Press.

Duncan, G. 1984. Years of Poverty, Years of Plenty. Ann Arbor: Institute for Social Research, University of Michigan.

Featherman, D., and R. Lerner. 1985. Ontogenesis and sociogenesis: Problematics for theory and research about development and socialization over the lifespan. American Sociological Review 50: 659-676.

Finch, C. 1987. Environmental influences on the aging brain. Pp. 77-91 in Perspectives in Behavioral Medicine, M. W. Riley, J. Matarazzo, and A. Baum, eds. Hillsdale, N.J.: Lawrence Erlbaum Associates.

Finch, C., and E.L. Schneider. 1985. Handbook of the Biology of Aging, 2nd ed. New York: Van Nostrand Reinhold.

George, L. K. 1989. Social and economic factors in geriatric psychiatry. Pp. 203-234 in Geriatric Psychiatry, E. Busse and D. Blazer, eds. Washington, D.C.: American Psychiatric Press.

Guilford, D. M. ed. 1988. The Aging Population in the Twenty-first Century. Washington, D.C.: National Academy Press.

Hagestad, G. 1987. Family. Pp. 247-249 in Encyclopedia of Aging, G. Maddox, ed. New York: Springer Publishing.

Hogan, D. P. 1985. The demography of life-span transitions: Temporal and gender comparisons. Pp. 65-80 in Gender and the Life Course, A. Rossi, ed. New York: Aldine.

Horowitz, A. 1985. Family caregiving to the frail elderly. Pp. 194-246 in Annual Review of Gerontology and Geriatrics, P. Lawton and G. Maddox, eds. New York: Springer Publishing.

Institute of Medicine. 1981. Airline Pilot Age, Health and Performance: Scientific and Medical Considerations. Washington, D.C.: National Academy Press.

Jensen, T. S., I. K. Genefke, N. Hyldebrandt, H. Pedersen, H. D. Petersen, and B. Weile. 1982. Cerebral atrophy in young torture victims. New England Journal of Medicine 307:1341-1344.

Katz, S., L. Branch, M. Branson, J. Papsiders, J. Beck, and D. Greer. 1983. Active life expectancy. New England Journal of Medicine 309:1218-1224.

Keith, J. 1985. Age in anthropological research. Pp. 232-263 in Handbook of Aging and the Social Sciences, R. Binstock and E. Shanas, eds. New York: Van Nostrand Reinhold.

Maddox, G. 1987a. Aging differently. The Gerontologist 27:557-564.

Maddox, G. 1987b. Psychosocial perspectives on aging. Pp. 15-28 in Perspectives in Behavioral Medicine: The Aging Dimension, M. Riley, J. Matarazzo, and A. Baum, eds. Hillsdale, N.J.: Lawrence Erlbaum Associates.

Maddox, G. and R. Campbell. 1985. Scope, concepts, and methods in the study of aging. Pp. 331 in Handbook of Aging and the Social Sciences, R. Binstock and E. Shanas, eds. New York: Van Nostrand Reinhold.

Manton, K. 1988. Planning long-term care for heterogeneous older populations. Pp. 217-257 in Varieties of Aging: Annual Review of Gerontology and Geriatrics, vol. 8, G. Maddox and P. Lawton, eds. New York: Springer Publishing.

Minkler, M., and R. Stone. 1983. The feminization of poverty and older women. The Gerontologist 25:351-357.

Moos, R. 1974. Evaluating Treatment Environments: A Social Ecological Approach. New York: John Wiley and Sons.

Moos, R. 1980. Specialized living arrangements for older people: A conceptual framework for evaluation. Journal of Social Issues 36:75-94.

Myers, G. 1985. Aging and worldwide population change. Pp. 173-198 in Handbook of Aging and the Social Sciences, R. Binstock and E. Shanas, eds. New York: Van Nostrand Reinhold.

Oppenheimer, V. 1982. Work and the Family: A Study in Social Demography. New York: Academic Press.

Riley, M. W., ed. 1988. Social Change and the Life Course, vols. 1 and 2. Beverly Hills, Calif.: Sage.

Riley, M. W., J. Matarazzo, and A. Baum, eds. 1987. Perspectives in Behavioral Medicine: The Aging Dimension. Hillsdale, N.J.: Lawrence Erlbaum Associates.

Rockstein, M., and M. Sussman. 1979. Biology and Aging. Belmont, Calif.: Wadsworth.

Rodin, J. 1986. Aging and health. Effects of the sense of control. Science 233:1271-1276.

Rodin, J., C. Timko, and B. Harris. 1985. The construct of control: Biological and psychological correlates. Pp. 3-55 in Annual Review of Gerontology and Geriatrics, vol. 5, P. Lawton and G. Maddox, eds. New York: Springer Publishing.

Rodin, J., C. Schooler, and K. W. Schaie, eds. 1990. Self-Directedness and Efficacy: Causes and Effects Throughout the Life Course. Hillsdale, N.J.: Lawrence Erlbaum Associates.

Schaie, K. W., and C. Schooler, eds. 1989. Social Structures and Aging: Psychological Processes. Hillsdale, N.J.: Lawrence Erlbaum Associates.

Schaie, K. W., and S. Willis. 1986. Can decline in intellectual functioning be reversed? Developmental Psychology 22:223-232.

Schooler, C., and K. W. Schaie, eds. 1987. Cognitive Functions and Social Structure over the Life Span. New York: A.B. Liss.

Siegler, I. and P. Costa. 1985. Health-behavior relationships. Pp. 144-166 in Handbook of the Psychology of Aging, 2nd ed., J. Birren and K. W. Schaie, eds. New York: Van Nostrand Reinhold.

Spenner, K. 1988. Social stratification, work, and personality. Annual Review of Sociology 14:69-97.

Sterns, H., and R. Alexander. 1987. Industrial gerontology: The aging individual and work. Pp. 243-264 in Annual Review of Gerontology and Geriatrics, vol. 7, W. Schaie, ed. New York: Springer Publishing.

Sussman, M. 1985. The family life of older people. Pp. 415-449 in Handbook of Aging and the Social Sciences, R. Binstock and E. Shanas, eds. New York: Van Nostrand Reinhold.

Torrey, B., K. Kinsella, and C. Taeuber. 1987. An Aging World. Washington, D.C.: Bureau of the Census, Department of Commerce.

Verbrugge, L. 1985. Gender and health: An update on hypotheses and evidence. Journal of Health and Social Behavior 26:157-177.

Verbrugge, L. 1988. Unveiling higher morbidity for men. Pp. 138-150 in Social Change and the Life Course, vol. 1, M. Riley ed. Beverly Hills, Calif.: Sage.

Woodruff-Pak, D. 1988. Psychology and Aging. New York: Prentice Hall.

Zarit, S. H. In press. Psychological aspects of aging and vision impairment. In Handbook on Aging and Vision, S. Timmerman and R. Kaarlela, eds. New York: American Foundation for the Blind.

5

Health Services Delivery Research

The existing health care system is fraught with problems for older persons and is best described as chaotic—disorganized, inadequate, and poorly distributed. There are major gaps separating acute and chronic care of older patients, and there is no organized array of services to meet these patients' chronic care needs or to provide for continuity of care. Equally, the health care system lacks the sensitivity to respond to the changing needs of individual older persons as they experience transitions in health. Although this report focuses on the health needs of the geriatric population, it must not be forgotten that many of the defects in long-term and chronic care apply to younger adults as well.

In the 1990s health care services will continue to be challenged by the changing demands imposed by the projected growth of the older population and especially by the growth of the "oldest old"—those persons 85 years of age and older who are most vulnerable to the problems of ill health and dependency. The growth of the older population will accelerate even more at the beginning of the next century as the baby-boom generation ages. Older persons consume an enormous amount of health services. Over the next decade those persons 80 years of age or older will likely become the largest single federal entitlement group, consuming $82.8 billion annually, including social security and other benefits (Torrey, 1985). Unfortunately, the response to this growing challenge has been far from adequate.

For example, the rate of production of health professionals (including those in health services delivery) is far short of the goals to provide care for dependent and chronically ill older persons and to meet future needs (National Institute on Aging, 1987). This deficiency will be compounded further by the loss of informal supports as more and more women join the labor force, therefore making them less available to provide care for older relatives.

Three trends are likely to influence health policy and health services for older persons in the 1990s: (1) the continuing problem of rising health care costs, (2) the growing concern with quality of care and cost-benefit ratios, and (3) the continuing rapid structural change of the health care service delivery system (Gilford, 1988).

Health services research focuses on broadening the knowledge base required to understand and influence the organization, delivery, and financing of health services to older persons. This research area cuts across the other four agenda areas in this report, relying heavily on knowledge from basic research in the biological and psychosocial arenas and linking with clinical research in studies designed to test delivery strategies for proven interventions in a variety of settings. By studying and making more effective the factors that influence delivery of health care to older individuals, research in health services delivery can contribute to decreasing disability and chronic illness, and to improving the quality of life of the older generation.

The following issues in health services delivery were identified by the committee as having greatest relevance to the research priorities listed in the next section:

- long-term care and continuity of care for older persons;
- financing health care for older persons;
- drug use and mental health services for older persons; and
- disability/disease prevention and health promotion services for older persons.

Implicit in research involving these areas are questions regarding (1) the extent to which functional status and/or quality of life for older persons is improved with various treatment options and (2) the efficacy and cost of care. This focus on effectiveness, outcome, and functional independence fits well with the new direction being taken by federal research centers.

An extended discussion of the issues related to health services research in aging appears in the Health Services Delivery Research Liaison Team report (see Appendix B).

LONG-TERM CARE AND CONTINUITY OF CARE FOR OLDER PERSONS

While there remain many unanswered questions concerning health services research related to older persons, the most pressing are those involving continuity of care, particularly with respect to long-term care. The objectives of long-term care are to help older persons cope with their disabilities, decrease dependence on others, and narrow the gap between actual and potential functioning (U.S. Department of Health and Human Services, 1980). Our system for delivering and financing long-term care is in an embryonic developmental state. A majority of the long-term care needs of this population are unmet or met by families (particularly the female spouse or daughters of the disabled older person), clearly indicating the need for governmental support of these important caregivers.

Long-term care is defined in a number of ways. The Health Care Financing Administration, the major federal agency involved in payment for long-term care for older persons, defines it as follows: "Long-term care refers to health, social and residential services provided to chronically disabled persons over an extended period of time. The need for long-term care is not necessarily identified with a particular diagnosis, but rather physical or mental disabilities that impair function in activities of daily living" (Doty et al., 1985).

A second definition can be found in the introduction to the Long-term Health Care Minimum Data Set: "Long-term health care refers to the professional or personal services required on a recurring or continuous basis by an individual because of chronic or permanent physical or mental impairment. These services may be provided in a variety of settings including the client's home" (U.S. Department of Health and Human Services, 1980). These and other definitions of long-term care (Kane and Kane, 1987) share two common elements: (1) the care continues over an extended period of time and provides varying degrees of intensity and resource deployment; (2) it is provided to persons who have lost (or never had) the capacity to care for themselves because of a chronic physical or mental illness or condition (Gilford, 1988).

The transition between acute and long-term care is complicated because the mechanisms that provide continuity of care for patients moving between acute and long-term care are not well developed. Consequently, issues surrounding continuity of care continue to plague older persons, their families, health care providers, and researchers.

Characteristics of Older Persons Requiring Long-Term Care

As noted in the Executive Summary and Recommendations for Funding, chronic diseases have become major contributors to death and disability among older persons in this country. However, the Panel for Statistics for an Aging Population (Gilford, 1988) states that "the diagnostic description of a person is seldom an indicator of his or her need for or utilization of long-term care because diagnosis alone gives no clue to how well or how poorly an individual functions. As a result, descriptions of behavior, rather than conditions, are used to describe the long-term care population."

About 20 percent of those 65 years of age and older need assistance to carry out some basic functions of adult life (LaPlante, 1988; Rice and LaPlante, 1988). Because of the dramatic and varied effect of age on disability, morbidity, and mortality, and because the older population is a widely heterogeneous group, investigators have suggested dividing this population into age subgroups. Gilford (1988), for instance, recommends three subgroups for health research purposes: the young-old (65 to 74 years), the old (75 to 84 years), and the oldest-old (85 years of age and over). This last group is most vulnerable to disability and the problems associated with ill health and frailty, and is most in need of long-term care services.

Data collection related to the natural history of chronic illness and disability, functional status, behavioral problems, and quality of life should be supported and expanded, with particular attention paid to changing cohorts (one-third of the membership in the aged population changes every 5 years). The recent mandate to collect functional status data on nursing home residents will provide a needed database on that population. Much more research is needed to elucidate the characteristics of special populations of older persons requiring long-term care. For example, little is known about how ethnic and class differences influence the need for or access to care.

Informal Providers of Long-Term Care

Family members and friends provide over 80 percent of all long-term care for older persons. Most caregivers are women; about 60 percent are 65 years old or older. More than 40 percent of those giving care rate their health as fair or poor, and over a third rate their health as poor or near poor (Stone et al., 1987).

The past decade of research indicates that family caregiving is a complex phenomenon. Tremendous variability exists in the nature of the care provided by family members, the stress and rewards related to that care on the part of the caregiver and older person, and the relationship between the formal and informal systems of care. Caregiving can be stressful for the caregiver and other family members (Zarit et al., 1986). In fact, recent research has shown that family members of older persons suffering from mental health problems are at risk for developing their own mental disorders (National Institute of Mental Health, 1988).

Those family members providing care to older family members receive little help from the formal health care system, for policymakers are concerned that extending publicly supported services to caregiving families might reduce the amount of family care provided to older persons. However, available evidence in this area suggests the opposite: the addition of formal services to a family caregiving situation does *not* reduce the amount of informal help provided to the older person (Stephens and Christianson, 1986).

Although our understanding of the phenomenon of family caregiving is increasing, we lack knowledge regarding caregiving among special populations (e.g., minority elderly persons, low-income elderly persons, elderly persons living alone), appropriate interventions for caregivers, and targeting interventions for this group (Brody, 1990). The nation depends on the family to provide most long-term care services in the community, but the knowledge base regarding how to assist family caregivers is inadequate.

Formal Long-Term Care

Organized long-term care in this country has been criticized as expensive, inadequate, disorganized, and biased toward institutional care (Harrington et al., 1985; Kane and Kane, 1987). The continuity of care between acute and long-term care is not well developed and often nonexistent (Estes, 1988).

During the past decade, attempts have been made to address these problems in long-term care. Results of these long-term care demonstrations (e.g., the channeling experiments) are difficult to interpret because of methodological problems encountered in the studies, but the hope that high-quality long-term care could be paid for with dollars recouped from the prevention of hospital care was not realized (Weissert et al., 1988).

Several criticisms have been directed at past long-term care experiments: (1) they failed to account for the complex and changing nature of long-term care needs; (2) the outcome measures used to evaluate such interventions were inappropriate; and (3) criteria for the selection of persons receiving such interventions were not appropriate. Results of long-term care demonstrations, however, do suggest an avenue for further research: both the conceptualization of long-term care and the methods used to study the efficacy of such services need to be reviewed. In addition, management mechanisms, such as case management, that are designed to facilitate continuity of care need to be evaluated.

Supply of Personnel for Long-Term Care

As our population ages, institutional and community-based long-term care systems are and will continue to be confronted with increasing numbers of older persons. Without intervention the recruitment, training, motivation, and reward of a competent work force to meet this population's service needs will continue to be insufficient. To a great degree this problem represents an economic and personnel issue, not a research question. The central questions are the following: Who should provide long-term care, and how can we pay the providers? To the extent that research can elucidate underlying factors affecting the choice of long-term care careers, work satisfaction, job design, and other work force-related matters, it should be supported.

Since long-term care providers are generally women, many are also poor and many are members of minority groups. From the provider's perspective the issues confronting workers in long-term care settings are "women's issues"—poor salaries and benefits, low job security, and lack of flexibility in scheduling. In many states, in fact, nonprofessional providers of long-term care are paid no better than the minimum wage.

Additionally, the gerontological and long-term care content of traditional physician, nurse, and social worker educational programs is inadequate (National Institute on Aging, 1987). Numerous professionals are involved in delivering health care to older persons; their roles, however, are not clearly defined. Research focusing on role definition and the costs and benefits of alternative long-term care providers should be undertaken. In order to avert a crisis within the next decade, research and demonstration programs that focus on the recruitment, training, retention, and quality of both nonprofessionals and professionals in long-term care are needed immediately.

Locus of Long-Term Care

At this point, little agreement exists about the most appropriate locus of long-term care. Is it the hospital, the home, the nursing home, or another long-term care facility? Research is needed to evaluate the attributes of each of these settings in relation to long-term care, the attributes of persons providing care within these settings, and the ability of specific settings to adjust to the changing needs and personal resources of older persons.

Quality Assurance

The interactions among the need for care (based on functional status), the nature of long-term care intervention, and the outcome of care are poorly understood. Lacking are standards for long-term care and valid and reliable measures of the need for and quality of care, including quality of care at different sites (e.g., home care), and instances where quality of care may conflict with quality of life. Development of such standards and measures for community-based care is particularly critical because of the shift in locus of care to the community. Such measures include indices of the quality of family care along with the quality of formal community care.

Several issues that cross health services and clinical research areas require attention. First, information about how a provider's perception of age and aging might affect treatment decisions in long-term care is essential. Second, research focusing on understanding rehabilitation strategies and their relationship to treatment outcomes is needed.

Technologies

Recent technical advances have the potential to enhance life for many disabled people, but little work has been done to delineate the positive and negative effects of such technologies. Three categories of technology are relevant to long-term care: (1) universal technologies (those shaping the environment in home and community to enhance, or to inhibit, independence), (2) individual technologies (those providing aids to individuals to help overcome deficits), and (3) life-sustaining technologies (those replacing or supplementing failed organs or bodily systems). The use of these technologies is value laden and leads to central questions that have not been addressed in our society. This and other ethical issues are discussed further in Chapter 6.

Theoretical development in the area of universal technologies suggests that such strategies may be key to reducing the need for both individual aids and service interventions (Orleans and Orleans, 1985; Zola, 1988). This area needs more research attention and represents a promising research direction.

FINANCING OF HEALTH CARE FOR OLDER PERSONS

Because of increased health care expenditures by federal and state governments and by individual older persons, health care financing has become one of the most critical issues to be addressed by the nation. Spending on health care services increased at an annual rate of 14.5 percent between 1977 and 1984 (Waldo and Lazenby, 1984) and has continued to increase since that time, but there is no evidence of a comparative improvement in health outcome. To a great degree, the methods used to finance health services govern both the nature of the services used by and available to older persons and the growth and development of the health and social service systems per se (Gilford, 1988).

Policymakers and health services researchers are confronted by five major issues related to the cost and financing of health care for older persons: (1) the continuing increase in the cost of health care despite efforts to restrain spending; (2) the highly concentrated distribution of health care expenses in which very few persons actually consume the majority of health care resources; (3) the individual and societal consequences of a health care policy that does not cover the costs of long-term care; (4) the impact of poverty on health status and access to care; and (5) the lack of suitable health care outcome measures.

These issues are complicated further by the fact that positive health is not distributed equally across society. Poverty negatively affects health; ill health impoverishes. Consequently, older persons most in need of health care are vulnerable not only because of ill health but also because of poverty. Since poverty is not distributed equally throughout the population but is more prevalent among women and members of minority groups, older persons who are poor, female, and members of a minority group are most vulnerable to the problems of illness.

These matters require research to help resolve the problems of health care financing for older persons. First, the factors that determine patterns of public and private health insurance arrangements for older persons must be understood. Of particular interest is the problem encountered by many older persons who have multiple insurance policies, overlapping or inadequate coverage, or health policies as part of the retirement benefits provided by government and industry. The failure of this fractured structure to protect many of the aged who are chronically ill stresses the urgency for intensive research on long-term care insurance for this vulnerable population. Second, the effects of financial barriers on access to and use of health services and on the health status of older persons must be better understood. Third, research related to the distribution of risk should be approached from a theoretical framework to guide definition and selection of risk factors and data collection. At present, models are tested using data that may not be appropriate. For example, investigators limited by inadequate research support have been forced to use data collected earlier by Medicare; these data often fail to identify the presence or absence of family caregivers or other supports for older persons. More work is needed to examine how financing and regulations shape the care system (by providing incentives for sites and types of care) and how Medicare policies influence screening and preventive services for older clients. Research should be directed toward better understanding providers who demonstrate inappropriate responses to older persons. Finally, more study is needed of careers in chronic care and of the cost of different levels and patterns of chronic care.

DRUG USE

Whereas persons 65 years old and over comprise about 12 percent of the U.S. population, they receive about 25 percent of the total number of prescriptions dispensed, and they account for about 30 percent of annual U.S. prescription drug expenditures. Three major and well-founded concerns arise in the area of geriatric drug use: inappropriate physician prescribing, widespread elderly patient noncompliance with drug regimens, and increasing drug prices.

Inappropriate Prescribing

Our body of knowledge regarding the effects of aging on drug therapy and drug metabolism is extensive (Bender, 1974; Lamy, 1984; Lipton and Lee, 1988; Montamat et al., 1989). However, increasing evidence indicates that prescribers do not follow the guidelines set forth in this research. Thus, a number of problems arise in the process of prescribing: a drug may be ordered when no drug is needed, or a prescription may be made for the wrong drug, a suboptimal drug, the incorrect dosage, or a dosage without knowledge of other medications being taken.

Evidence of geriatric prescribing problems can be found in the high rate of drug-related hospitalizations among older people. Among all patients admitted to the hospital, patients 65 years old and older have the highest admission rates (10 to 25 percent) for drug-induced symptoms, and this problem appears not to have changed significantly during the past decade (Levy et al., 1979; Bergman and Wilholm,

1981; Ives et al., 1987). Recent studies focusing on geriatric patients suggest that 10 to 31 percent of hospital admissions are associated with drug-related problems (Williamson and Chopin, 1980; Popplewell and Henschke, 1982; Grymonpre et al., 1988). Drug-induced hospitalizations are associated with appreciable morbidity and mortality; the cost of such hospital care is estimated at $4.5 to $7 billion annually (Kusserow, 1989).

Although most of the studies identify specific drug classes implicated in drug admissions, they do not identify the specific reasons the drugs are associated with the problem. For example, if a given drug is responsible for a hospital admission, is the problem related to drug dosage, drug schedule, drug allergy, drug duplication, drug-drug interaction, or drug selection? Additional research is needed to add to our understanding of the mechanisms through which specific drugs lead to problems associated with hospitalization. We also need to learn more about the incidence of prescribing problems among older persons living in the community. The cumulative burden of drug-related morbidity among elderly outpatients may have enormous clinical and economic consequences.

Noncompliance

Older persons are more likely than younger persons to misuse medications (Cooper et al., 1978; Lamy, 1984; Darnell et al., 1986). A systematic investigation of communication among patients and providers should be undertaken to assess the extent to which good communication enhances compliance on the part of older persons (Lipton and Lee, 1988). Systems of information retrieval for physicians, pharmacists, and other providers should be developed and evaluated. Finally, demonstrations are needed to test approaches to improve compliance by older populations.

Because the aging process alters pharmacodynamics and pharmacokinetics, older persons are at risk for untoward drug effects (Law and Chalmers, 1976; Kiernan and Isaacs, 1981). In addition, many older persons with multiple chronic illnesses take more than one drug, increasing the chance of an adverse drug reaction (Steel et al., 1981; Hutchinson et al., 1986). While we know that older persons are at risk for drug reactions for several reasons, we do not know the extent to which older persons are at risk. Work by Lipton and Lee (1988) identifies multiple strategies to reduce these risks through such broad-based interventions as modified labeling and simplified drug schedules.

Drug Costs and Older Persons

National expenditures for "drugs and medical sundries"—a category that includes prescription and nonprescription drugs and medical supplies dispensed through retail channels—accounted for almost 7 percent of health spending or $34 billion in 1987. Drug costs totaled about $9 billion for older persons that year.

The number of drugs prescribed increases with age, and the average price of prescriptions also rises with age. Overall, older persons pay 14 percent more per prescription than do those under age 65. It is important to note that older persons are not being charged more for their medications. Rather, they take a different mix of drugs, and their prescriptions extend over a long-term, not acute, treatment period. Because they use more drugs and pay higher prices for prescriptions than do younger patients, older patients are more likely than other age groups to incur high drug costs. They are also more likely to pay a higher percentage of out-of-pocket expenses for drugs.

What about the demographic distribution of drug expenses incurred by older persons? Results of a 1980 national survey revealed that the proportion of prescription drug expenses reimbursed by private insurance was similar for both poor and near poor older persons: 7.7 percent and 10.7 percent, respectively. However, that statistic rises significantly—up to 20.6 percent—for those who are not poor. All three groups had out-of-pocket expenses of approximately half of the total costs of drugs. The near poor (those living in families whose income is above the poverty level but less than or equal to twice the poverty level) are particularly vulnerable to this out-of-pocket cost burden.

It is important to emphasize that this information was collected in 1980, before the escalation of drug prices. Since 1981, prescription drug prices have increased two to three times faster than all other consumer prices (Lipton and Lee, 1988). As a result, drug prices have become a source of growing concern for consumers, policymakers, and both individual and institutional purchasers. Although the real income of the aged poor and near poor has remained relatively static in recent years, with Social Security payments increasing at the same rate as inflation, the expenditure for drugs most likely has increased as the result of drug price inflation. Therefore, drug expenditures relative to income may be even greater now than at the time of the 1980 survey.

MENTAL HEALTH SERVICES

There is growing interest in the older person's use of mental health services, with some researchers noting that older persons seem to use fewer mental health services than do younger persons (German et al., 1985; Leaf et al., 1985; Borson et al., 1986; German et al., 1987; Goldstrom et al., 1987; Lurie and Swan, 1987). The need to understand the older person's use (or nonuse) of mental health services is important for several reasons: (1) the high incidence of dementia in the older population, (2) the high prevalence of mental impairment of older persons in nursing homes, and (3) the high prevalence of alcohol abuse or dependency among older persons admitted to county or state mental hospitals. In the community 10 to 25 percent of older persons have some degree of mental impairment. Among men, the incidence of suicide dramatically increases with age. In short, mental illness is common in older persons, but often is untreated. Research is needed to investigate how older persons use mental health services and why. Of particular interest are the effects of race, gender, and social status on service utilization.

Alzheimer's disease is widely recognized as the major mental health problem of the older population, but little is known about its epidemiology and treatment. Of particular interest is the delineation of risk factors associated with dementia. Depression is another common problem of late adulthood; yet because there is little agreement on the definition of this condition, depression in older people may not be recognized widely. From a health services perspective, innovative methods for the treatment of depression that are acceptable to older persons should be developed and evaluated.

Our understanding of the less common clinical problems of aging—schizophrenia, bipolar disease, and other psychotic conditions—is very limited. Research is needed to examine both those who develop a psychotic condition, such as paranoia, in older age and those who were diagnosed with such disorders earlier in life. Even where our knowledge base is firm, clinicians providing the bulk of services to older persons may not recognize the signs and symptoms of major mental illness.

Investigation is critically needed on mental illness in special populations of older persons. Little is known, for example, about the mental health status or needs of older persons who are members of minority groups. Of the older population, those who are institutionalized have the least understood but highest prevalence of mental disorders (National Institute of Mental Health, 1988). We do not know what services are available to this group, nor do we know what services are needed or how they should be financed. Research also is needed to elucidate the interactive processes among disability, disease, mental health, the environment, and the cost of health services. Such a holistic approach should lead to a better understanding of the panoply of services needed by older persons. Finally, research is required to elucidate the cost and outcomes of various patterns of mental health care. How well, for example, do community mental health centers meet the needs of older persons? These data should be related to the reimbursement system that currently does not pay for many types of mental health services.

DISABILITY/DISEASE PREVENTION AND HEALTH PROMOTION SERVICES

Although some work has been undertaken in the area of disease prevention through risk reduction,* there is still a crucial need for clinical research in this area. Lacking is consistent evidence regarding the effects of risk reduction on the presence of disease conditions; no systematic research has been undertaken on risk reduction in late adulthood. Lifestyle prescriptions for older populations are now based on research done on younger populations.

Several clinical research questions need to be answered before health services research can proceed:

- Are accepted risk factors for disease the same in direction and magnitude for older persons as they are for younger persons?
- What are the prevalence estimates for specific risk factors by demographics within the older population?
- Are interventions known to be effective with younger persons equally effective and acceptable in reducing risk in older people?
- Does the reduction of risk factors make any difference in the health status of older persons?
- What is the relationship between disease and disability?

If research does support the need for intervention, then demonstrations designed to deliver preventive services to older persons should be developed. Research also is needed to identify risk factors for disability; risk-reduction programs can then be developed and evaluated.

---

*See the Institute of Medicine's 1990 report, *The Second Fifty Years: Promoting Health and Preventing Disability* (Washington, D.C.: National Academy Press).

RESEARCH PRIORITIES

The committee identified five research priorities in the area of health services research. These priorities represent the broad areas within which specific research questions and proposals can be framed. It is noteworthy that the field of health services delivery, as with some aspects of clinical science and behavioral and social studies, offers opportunities for research in nursing and other aspects of health care that may contribute significantly to the field of investigation of aging.

- **The committee proposes that research be undertaken into long-term care and continuity of care for older persons.**

This priority area includes research into factors that determine the need for and use of long-term care services, questions regarding the organization and delivery of long-term care services, the special role of the family in the delivery of care, and the growing question of adapting modern technology to enhance the ability of older persons to live independently. Also included in this category is research into the nature of the hospital as an institution and the role of nursing facilities and health care institutions for the older person. Finally, this priority area includes research at three levels—the individual, the institution, and the society—that affect recruitment, training, and quality of providers of both formal and informal long-term care.

- **The committee recommends research on the cost and financing of health care in the older population.**

This priority area includes research into reducing financial barriers to care for older persons. Of particular interest are questions related to financing of insurance for older persons, most notably coverage for long-term care, mental health, rehabilitation, and disease prevention and health promotion services. Studies of outcome measures in this area also are important.

- **The committee recommends research on drug therapy in older persons.**

This priority area includes research into the factors influencing the development and regulatory approval of drugs and the effectiveness and efficiency of prescribing, dispensing, and taking pharmaceuticals. Equally, research should be undertaken into drug-related phenomena that affect the social and physical functioning of older persons.

- **The committee recommends research on mental health services in the older population.**

This priority area includes research into the factors that determine the need for and use of mental health services, the role of treatment for mental illness as a factor in improving the social and physical functioning of older persons, and the effect of early life treatment in reducing later-life disability from mental disorders.

- **The committee recommends research on disability/disease prevention and health promotion in older persons.**

This priority area includes research into developing new models for the delivery of appropriate behavior change programs for elderly populations.

ADDITIONAL RESEARCH OPPORTUNITIES

The committee considers the preceding five research priorities to be the most critical. Additional important opportunities in health services delivery research include research into alternative methods of delivering long-term care, including models that focus on a particular subgroup (e.g., posthospital management) and that provide linkage of housing arrangements with community long-term care facilities; research to examine the effect of employer-initiated cost sharing on the use of preventive and treatment services by older persons; research on the effect of interventions to reduce the incidence of inappropriate drug treatment decisions by physicians; research to study the provision of mental health services to elderly institutionalized persons in the context of need, utility, and outcome; and research to investigate and compare the relative contribution of accepted risk factors in the development of disease among young and aged populations.

RESOURCES REQUIRED

The committee recommends increased support over current health services research spending during the next 5 years for increased funding of research, for construction, for training, for the expansion of infrastructure (databases, library support, computer capability), and for the addition of new Centers of Excellence in Geriatric and Gerontological Research and Training (Claude Pepper Centers). Funding needs are described in greater detail in the Executive Summary and Recommendations for Funding. Specifically, increased funding in age-related research is recommended in order to raise the number of approved grants that are funded from less than one in four (24 percent) to one in two. In addition to the dollars for research activities, funds are needed to support a minimum of 140 additional predoctoral and postdoctoral fellowships per year for training in health services research careers, for specific infrastructure needs, and for construction costs. Health services research also will participate in the added funds for support of programs of geriatric and gerontological research that are located within current medical centers (administrative locus, as compared with geographically established centers).

CROSS-DISCIPLINARY AND CROSSCUTTING ISSUES

Most of the research priorities identified in this chapter cross disciplinary lines, focusing on issues that benefit from clinical, behavioral, and social science as well as health services research. Beyond that, four key crosscutting issues must be addressed directly.

First, an understanding of the effects of gender, class, and ethnicity is salient to every priority area listed in this chapter. Second, ethical issues that must be thoughtfully analyzed and researched are embedded in each priority. Third, save in specific areas, health services research in the area of health promotion/disease prevention cannot proceed until clinical research provides clear mechanisms for risk reduction in the older age groups. This need has been identified by Lipton and Lee (1988) who state with respect to drug use research:

> Despite the existence of a great deal of information regarding drug therapy and older patients (especially information gathered in recent years), there is a need for more research. Areas requiring further study include the nature of age-related biological, physiological and pathological changes; ways in which these changes affect the elderly person's response to drugs; and the kinds of drug prescribing, dispensing, and administration appropriate to deal with these changes. An area that has remained virtually unexamined involves the psychological changes (e.g., depression) and social changes (e.g., loss of spouse) that accompany aging and the way they affect the older person's need for, use of, and response to drugs. Drug epidemiology studies—large-scale studies of drug use and its relationship to clinical outcomes—are urgently needed in elderly populations, especially with regard to psychotropic agents. Private foundations and federal funding agencies (particularly the National Institutes of Health and the Alcohol, Drug Abuse and Mental Health Administration) should give these areas high priority on their agendas.

Fourth, the dynamic nature of both the aging process and the health care delivery system means that there is a great need for longitudinal research. Most of the research areas in this section can best be addressed using this approach. Longitudinal research is complicated by a series of predictable methodological and situational issues that must be taken into account when planning for resources in this area.

REFERENCES

Bender, A. D. 1974. Pharmacodynamic principles of drug therapy in the aged. Journal of the American Geriatrics Society 22:296-303.

Bergman, U., and B. E. Wilholm. 1981. Drug-related problems causing admission to a medical clinic. European Journal of Clinical Pharmacology 20:193-200.

Borson, S., R. A. Barnes, W. A. Kukull, J. T. Okimoto, R. C. Veith, T. S. Inui, W. Carter, and M. A. Raskind. 1986. Symptomatic depression in elderly medical outpatients. 1. Prevalence, demography, and health service utilization. Journal of the American Geriatrics Society 34:341-347.

Brody, E. 1990. Women in the Middle. New York: Springer Publishing.

Cooper, J. W., and C. G. Bagwell. 1978. Contribution of the consultant pharmacist to rational drug usage in the long-term facility. Journal of the American Geriatrics Society 26:513-520.

Darnell, J. C., M. D. Murray, B. L. Martz, and M. Weinberger. 1986. Medication use by ambulatory elderly: An in-home survey. Journal of the American Geriatrics Society 34:1-4.

Doty, P., K. Liu, and J. Weiner. 1985. Special report: An overview of long-term care. Health Care Financing Review 6:69-78.

Estes, C. 1988. Cost-containment and the elderly: Conflict or challenge? Journal of the American Geriatrics Society 36:68-72.

German, P. S., S. Shapiro, and E. A. Skinner. 1985. Mental health of the elderly: Use of health and mental health services. Journal of the American Geriatrics Society 33:246-252.

German, P. S., S. Shapiro, E. A. Skinner, M. Von Korff, L. E. Klein, R. W. Turner, M. L. Teitelbaum, J. Burke, and B. J. Burns. 1987. Detection and management of mental health problems of older patients by primary care providers. Journal of the American Medical Association 257:489-493.

Gilford, D. M. 1988. The Aging Population in the Twenty-first Century. Washington, D.C.: National Academy Press.

Goldstrom, I. D., B. J. Burns, L. G. Kessler, M. A. Feuerberg, D. B. Larson, N. E. Miller, and W. J. Cromer. 1987. Mental health services use by elderly adults in a primary care setting. Journal of Gerontology 42:147-153.

Grymonpre, R. E., P. A. Mitenko, D. S. Sitar, F. Y. Aoke, and P. R. Montgomery. 1988. Drug-associated hospital admissions in older medical patients. Journal of the American Geriatrics Society 36:1094-1098.

Harrington, C., R. J. Newcomer, and C. L. Estes. 1985. Long Term Care of the Elderly: Public Policy Issues. Beverly Hills, Calif.: Sage.

Hutchinson, T. A., M. M. Flegel, M. S. Kramer, D. G. Leduc, and H. H. Kong. 1986. Frequency, severity, and risk factors for adverse reactions in adult outpatients: A prospective study. Journal of Chronic Disease 39:533-542.

Ives, T. J., E. J. Bentz, and R. E. Gwyther. 1987. Drug-related admissions to a family medicine inpatient service. Archives of Internal Medicine 147:1117-1120.

Kane, R. A., and R. L. Kane. 1987. Long-Term Care: Principles, Programs and Policies. New York: Springer Publishing.

Kiernan, P. J., and J. B. Isaacs. 1981. Use of drugs by the elderly. Journal of the Royal Society of Medicine 74:196-200.

Kusserow, R. P. 1989. Medicare Drug Utilization Review. Washington, D.C.: Office of the Inspector General.

Lamy, P. P. 1984. Hazards of drug use in the elderly. Postgraduate Medicine 76:50-53, 56-57, 60-61.

LaPlante, M. 1988. Data on Disability from the National Health Interview Survey, 1983-1984. Report 88-P-6, prepared with InfoUse. Washington, D.C.: National Institute on Disability and Rehabilitation Research.

Law, R., and C. Chalmers. 1976. Medicines and elderly people: A general practice survey. British Medical Journal 1(609):565-568.

Leaf, P. J., M. M. Livingston, G. L. Tischler, M. M. Weissman, C. E. Holzer III, and J. K. Myers. 1985. Contact with health professionals for the treatment of psychiatric and emotional problems. Medical Care 23:1322-1337.

Levy, M., M. Lipshitz, and M. Eliakim. 1979. Hospital admissions due to adverse drug reactions. American Journal of Medicine 39:49-56.

Lipton, H. P., and P. R. Lee. 1988. Drugs and the Elderly: Clinical, Social and Policy Perspectives. Stanford, Calif.: Stanford University Press.

Lurie, E. E., and J. H. Swan. 1987. Serving the Mentally Ill Elderly: Problems and Perspectives. Lexington, Mass.: Lexington/Heath.

Montamat, S. C., B. J. Cusack, and R. E. Vestal. 1989. Management of drug therapy in the elderly. New England Journal of Medicine 321:303-309.

National Institute of Mental Health. 1988. Research and Activities Report of the Mental Disorders of the Aging Research Branch (mimeo). Rockville, Md.

National Institute on Aging. 1987. Personnel for health needs of the elderly through year 2020. In Administrative Document of the U.S. Department of Health and Human Services. Washington, D.C.: U.S. Government Printing Office.

Orleans, M., and P. Orleans. 1985. High and low technology: Sustaining life at home. International Journal of Technology Assessment in Health Care 1:353-364.

Popplewell, P. Y., and P. J. Henschke. 1982. Acute admissions to a geriatric assessment unit. Medical Journal of Australia 1:343-344.

Rice, D. P., and M. LaPlante. 1988. Chronic illness, disability, and increasing longevity. Pp. 5-55 in The Economics and Ethics of Long-Term Care and Disability, S. Sullivan and M. E. Lewin, eds. Washington, D.C.: American Enterprise Institute for Public Policy Research.

Steel, K., P. M. Gertman, C. Creszeni, and J. Anderson. 1981. Iatrogenic illness on a general medical service at a university hospital. New England Journal of Medicine 304:638-642.

Stephens, S. A., and J. B. Christianson. 1986. Informal Care of the Elderly. Lexington, Mass.: Lexington Books.

Stone, R., G. L. Cafferata, and J. Sangl. 1987. Caregivers of frail elderly. The Gerontologist 27:616-626.

Torrey, B. 1985. Sharing increasing costs on declining income: The visible dilemma of the invisible aged. Milbank Memorial Fund Quarterly; Health and Society 63:377-394.

U.S. Department of Health and Human Services. 1980. Report of the National Committee on Vital and Health Statistics. Long-Term Health Care Minimum Data Set. DHHS Pub, No. (PHS)80-1158. Hyattsville, Md.: Office of Health Research, Statistics, and Technology, National Center for Health Statistics.

Waldo, D., and H. Lazenby. 1984. Demographic characteristics and health care use and expenditures by the aged in the U.S.: 1972–1984. Health Care Financing Review 6:1-29.

Weissert, W. G., C. M. Cready, and J. E. Pawelak. 1988. The past and future of home- and community-based long-term care. Milbank Memorial Fund Quarterly; Health and Society 66:309-388.

Williamson, J., and J. M. Chopin. 1980. Adverse reactions to prescribed drugs in the elderly: A multicenter investigation. Age and Ageing 9:73-80.

Zarit, S. H., P. A. Todd, and J. M. Zarit. 1986. Subjective burden of husbands and wives as caregivers: A longitudinal study. The Gerontologist 26:260-266.

Zola, I. K. 1988. Policies and programs concerning aging and disability: Toward a unifying agenda. Pp. 90-130 in The Economics and Ethics of Long-Term Care and Disability, S. Sullivan and M. E. Lewin, eds. Washington, D.C.: American Enterprise Institute for Public Policy Research.

6

Research in Biomedical Ethics

Individual older persons and the aging American society as a whole face dilemmas regarding life-sustaining treatment, distribution of limited health care resources, and participation in clinical research by vulnerable elderly persons. Research can help clarify the underlying ethical issues, analyze the arguments for and against various stances, and forge a social consensus to guide clinical care and overall health care policy. Furthermore, empirical studies in biomedical ethics can help identify in current practice any variance from recommended guidelines, and develop guidelines and evaluate interventions to improve clinical practice.

Although the topics and research recommendations developed in this chapter focus on the problems of older persons, many of these issues (e.g., decreased mental competence, need for advance directives, disabled patients without families or friends) concern younger disabled persons as well.

RESEARCH PRIORITIES

Sufficient funds should be made available to conduct research on the ethical dilemmas involved in the provision of life-sustaining treatment, the allocation of health care resources, and the participation in clinical research by frail and elderly persons. Using the broad areas of investigation listed here, one can formulate specific research questions to include both empirical and analytical studies.

Life-Sustaining Treatment in Older Persons

- **The committee recommends research on decisions regarding life-sustaining treatment in older persons.**

The medical technology that allows physicians to prolong life in patients with serious illnesses may not always be appropriate. According to ethical, medical, and legal guidelines, competent informed patients may refuse life-sustaining treatments. For patients who lack the capacity to give informed consent or refusal, such as elderly patients with severe dementia, decisions concerning medical care should respect wishes previously expressed by the patient (President's Commission for the Study of Ethical Problems in Medicine and Biomedical and Behavioral Research, 1982, 1983; Annas and Glantz, 1986a; American College of Physicians, 1989a,b). Such declarations by competent patients of what care they would or would not want if they became incompetent are called "advance directives." However, these guidelines may be problematic for elderly persons. Although most elderly persons welcome the opportunity to discuss their preferences for (or against) life-sustaining treatment, they infrequently develop or invoke specific advance directives (Lo et al., 1986).

Further knowledge is needed about ethical questions concerning both those isolated elderly patients who are institutionalized and those older persons who are not institutionalized, but who do not have relatives or close friends to act as surrogates. (It is important to note that the number of isolated older people most likely will continue to grow in the coming decades.)

Improving Discussions About Life-Sustaining Treatment

Research is required to lay the foundation for increased understanding of what requires improvement in decisions about life-sustaining treatment among physicians, families, and institutions. Educational interventions that encourage health care providers and patients to discuss life-sustaining treatments need to be developed. In the absence of explicit discussions, physicians and family members cannot predict a patient's preferences for (or against) treatment (Bedell and Delbanco, 1984; Uhlmann et al., 1988). Such discussions might be more effective if more were known about how physicians currently engage in them. More needs to be known about how well elderly patients understand the issues at stake, how their understanding might be improved, how their preferences might change over time, and how they can be given specific directives about life-sustaining treatments.

The focus of research on older patients' acceptance or rejection of life-sustaining treatment may vary, depending on whether the decision involves patients and their families or is limited to isolated institutionalized and noninstitutionalized older persons.

Several problems with advance directives must be resolved. The durable power of attorney for health care is the most effective type of advance directive because it allows competent patients both to designate surrogates and to specify the types of treatments they do and do not want (President's Commission for the Study of Ethical Problems in Medicine and Biomedical and Behavioral Research, 1983; Buchanan and Brock, 1986; Force, 1988). However, such advance directives cannot be used by patients with no relatives or friends to be designated as surrogate decision makers. Living wills are ineffective for such patients because they apply only in cases of terminal illness and are inapplicable to such situations as severe dementia (President's Commission for the Study of Ethical Problems in Medicine and Biomedical and Behavioral Research, 1983; Buchanan and Brock, 1986; Force, 1988). Thus, to ensure that patients' preferences are respected if they become incompetent, new procedures need to be devised for patients with no one to serve as a surrogate. Because legal problems often arise in this context, as well as in other areas reviewed in this chapter, these problems present an opportunity for collaborative research between medical and legal scholars.

Improving Decision Making for Incompetent Patients Who Have Not Given Clear Advance Directives

Such situations are common and perplexing. Consensus has not been reached regarding either the level of specificity required by an advance directive or the discretion afforded family members in interpreting such directives (Veatch, 1984; Rhoden, 1988). Further, when the incompetent patient's preferences are unclear or unknown, no specific guidelines delineate how the patient's best interests should be determined, what role quality of life considerations should play, and what safeguards are desirable for particularly vulnerable nursing home residents (Buchanan and Brock, 1986; Lo and Dornbrand, 1986; Lo, 1988). In addition, research is indicated on how advance directives play out—behaviorally and legally—to inform revision in ethical standards and law. Further analysis of these issues is needed; discrepancies among clinical practice, ethical guidelines, and case law must be studied.

Defining the Role of Institutional Ethics Committees, Particularly Within Nursing Homes

Such committees have been proposed to improve decision making about life-sustaining treatments and to serve as an alternative to time-consuming and cumbersome legal proceedings (Cranford and Doudera, 1984). However, more must be learned about the benefits and drawbacks of such committees, their optimal structure and procedures, and their impact on clinical decisions (Lo, 1987).

Establishing Medical Futility

Physicians and other providers sometimes decide to withhold treatment because it is considered medically futile. Better data are needed on prognosis and outcome in seriously ill elderly patients. Although some good data are available about cardiopulmonary resuscitation (Bedell and Delbanco, 1984), many other life-sustaining treatments should be studied, particularly those affecting the critically ill and patients of very advanced age (over age 85) (Force, 1988). In addition, the concept of futility itself should be analyzed. The term can be used in many ways, some of which do not constitute acceptable justification for physicians to withhold treatment (Youngner, 1988).

Resolving Disagreements Between Health Care Professionals and Patients (or Patients' Families)

Caregivers may insist on giving a treatment—particularly artificial feedings—despite the refusal of the patient or family (Steinbrook and Lo, 1988; Miles et al., 1989). Court rulings on cases involving such disagreements are often misunderstood by physicians, such as interpreting the Supreme Court's ruling on nasogastric feedings in the Cruzan case to mean that nasogastric feedings can *never* be discontinued in incompetent patients (Kapp and Lo, 1986; Annas, 1990; Lo et al., 1990). Formal study should be undertaken to learn more about how physician perception of legal requirements and liability affects decision making, and further legal and ethical analyses are needed to begin to develop a consensus on how best to resolve these dilemmas. An area of research involving disagreements between caregivers and patients that deserves further attention, although it relates more to patient comfort and contentment than to life-and-death issues, involves study of day-to-day ethical problems, such as conflicts between autonomy and paternalism in long-term care (Kane and Caplan, 1989). Specific examples include nursing home patients who do not wish to have their hours of rising and retiring, along with other activities, set by caregivers, or who want to be able to refuse therapy, even when it is indicated.

Issues of Equity and Access

- **The committee recommends research on issues of equity and access.**

The projected increase in the number of elderly Americans, the rising costs of Medicare, competing social needs, and continuing federal budget deficits have imposed artificial pressures on caregivers to limit health care spending in general and to limit care to the elderly in particular (as seen, for example, in the early discharge and decreased rehabilitative care given to patients operated on for hip fracture). Although difficult decisions regarding allocation of scarce resources are inevitable, no agreement now exists on how such rationing may be accomplished in an equitable manner that does not compromise access to basic health care resources (Daniels, 1986; Engelhardt and Rie, 1986; Miller and Miller, 1986).

Identification of Criteria for Appropriate Practice Standards

Standards must be developed for such health care services as cataract surgery, hip replacement, and cancer screening and treatment for the elderly. Given the wide regional variation in the use of such treatments, it is important to develop criteria that establish when these treatments become appropriate. Health services research on functional outcomes can elucidate the effectiveness of various therapies and identify those groups of patients for whom certain therapies are less effective. In addition, public forums and consensus conferences that focus on resource allocation can seek to forge public and professional agreement on the priorities to be set among various therapies to be made available to different patient populations.

Age as a Criterion for Allocating Health Care Resources

Chronological age per se has been proposed as the basis upon which health care expenditures should be limited (Brook, 1989). However, critics point out that the elderly are heterogeneous in both function and prognosis and that justice requires that costly therapies used in other age groups also should be scrutinized (Avorn, 1984; Callahan, 1987; Schneider, 1989). More data, debate, and analysis are needed to determine if or when health care resources should be allocated on the basis of age and to define those basic health care resources to which all elderly persons should have access. No data concerning how the American public regards rationed care based on age have been amassed. It is important to identify misunderstandings of fact regarding rationing (e.g., that inordinate sums are spent on the intensive care of dying older patients) that might hinder policy decisions; educational programs must be devised to correct such misconceptions. Furthermore, the views of the public will be crucial in shaping a social consensus on these complicated and potentially divisive issues.

In addition to helping us determine how health care resources should be allocated, research can help us understand the current system of allocating health care services to the elderly (Avorn, 1984; Scitovsky and Capron, 1986; Anderson et al., 1989). For example, present incentives for early patient discharge, for outpatient in lieu of inpatient care, and for technological services rather than preventive and case management care may have particularly deleterious effects on the elderly (Grumet, 1989; Leaf, 1989). The distribution of benefits and burdens of the current allocation system should be examined, discussed, and debated more explicitly to facilitate more realistic decision making.

Allocation of Resources for Patient Care and for Research

Resources available to devote to biomedical research, health services research, and patient care research are not unlimited. As suggested throughout this report, priorities need to be set to allocate these limited resources in a rational manner. Until recently, little research was dedicated to the most prevalent and disabling diseases of old age—the degenerative neurological diseases and the musculoskeletal diseases. Wide-ranging discussion, both with members of the public at large (especially the elderly) and with scientists, could help clarify the value choices that must be made to set future research priorities and could help establish procedures and criteria for allocating resources to the research endeavor.

Other research issues concerning allocation of resources include decisions about distribution of funds to support preventive care versus high-technology care in older persons, the allocation of funds to support health education compared with direct health care, the competition among different age cohorts for expensive treatment programs (e.g., bone marrow and organ transplant, hemodialysis, coronary artery bypass surgery), and the assignment of research support to study the role of poverty in health among elderly persons as compared to younger subjects.

Ethical Issues in Aging Research

- **The committee recommends research on biomedical ethical issues involving participation in clinical research by frail elderly persons.**

This report documents the need for significant increases in research on diseases and disorders afflicting the elderly. Disorders such as dementia, incontinence, and falls impair functioning and may lead to either home-based or institutional long-term care. Paradoxically, frail elderly persons with such disorders—ideal research subjects— may be among those least likely or physically able to participate as subjects of research (Brieger, 1978; Annas and Glantz, 1986b; Dubler, 1987; Kane and Manoukian, 1989). However, intensive research is needed to elucidate the etiology of these conditions and to find effective treatments. Patients with severe dementia lack the capacity to give informed consent to participate in research. Institutionalization, regardless of cognitive function, *impairs the autonomy of residents*, making it difficult for them to decline to participate in research (Cassel, 1985, 1987, 1988). These problems were amply documented by the National Commission for the Protection of Human Subjects of Biomedical and Behavioral Research in 1974 and led to appropriate restraint in the use of nursing home patients as research subjects (National Commission for the Protection of Human Subjects of Biomedical and Behavioral Research, 1978a,b). For this vitally needed research, the population of incapacitated and institutionalized people able to serve as research subjects, including those *not* of geriatric age, must be expanded. How best to accomplish this goal is, itself, an important research question.

Innovative Approaches to Informed Consent

Researchers should develop and evaluate the use of simplified or alternative ways to inform patients about research projects (Levine, 1986). For example, videotapes might enable persons with mild to moderate dementia to understand enough about a research project to give informed consent (Cassel, 1987). Similarly, linguistic analysis of impaired language processing might help physicians communicate better with research-eligible patients suffering from mild dementia.

Proxy Consent for Incompetent Patients

Consent by a family member or a close friend may not meet the standard of substituted judgment, which states that the proxy has given consent or refusal as desired by the incapacitated subject (Tymchuck et al., 1988). Studies have shown that proxies often give consent based on their own value system, not that of the patient. Thus, the practice of obtaining consent from relatives of incapacitated patients needs to be reevaluated. Several methods to improve such substituted judgment should be considered, such as education of the public and, in particular, of relatives of patients eligible for research studies in the concept of proxy consent to research participation. Furthermore, educational interventions aimed at the elderly could encourage them to give advance directives for participating in research, just as they are encouraged to do for medical care decisions.

Institutional ethics committees might evaluate the appropriateness of a proxy's consent. In some situations, the appropriate standard for participation of incompetent patients in research might be that of the patient's best interests (Warren et al., 1986). Research and further discussion should disclose the specific situations in which the best-interest standard is most appropriate.

Attitudes Toward Participation in Research

Philosophers have posited that research should be a partnership between investigator and subject in which both parties understand the potential benefits to the patient and to the larger society (Fletcher et al., 1985; Veatch, 1987). However, some older people fear being research subjects (Faden and Beauchamp, 1986). Institutional safeguards are enacted based on the assumption that exploitation is possible, or even probable, without such protection. Thus, it becomes important to examine public attitudes about research. What responsibility does an ill person have to participate in research designed to understand and ameliorate conditions afflicting himself and others of a similar age? What discourages an elderly person from participating in research, and how might those barriers be overcome? Understanding how elderly people answer these questions would further our nation's sense of mission regarding research on aging.

Research Review in Long-Term Care

Although an increasing amount of research is being conducted in nursing homes, the process of review through institutional review boards (IRBs) remains sporadic and irregular (Ratzen, 1980). Nursing home and home care research affiliated with an academic center is generally reviewed by the center's IRB. However, such IRBs may not be knowledgeable about long-term care and may react in either an overprotective or an underprotective manner. Moreover, research lacking academic affiliation is being conducted increasingly in nursing homes and home care programs. In such cases, review of research may be ad hoc or totally lacking. In order to promote the quality of research, to educate investigators about the ethical dilemmas they face, and to protect research subjects, scientists should explore the establishment of community-based IRBs or other alternatives for review of methods used in research projects.

ADDITIONAL RESEARCH OPPORTUNITIES

The following topics provide additional research opportunities:

- treatment of older persons with experimental therapies that may involve increased risk to them, such as genetic engineering or organ transplants, which may raise ethical issues that require systematic study through research; and
- the trade-off between quality of care and quality of life for older patients.

CONCLUSIONS AND RESOURCE RECOMMENDATIONS

Ethical issues are an inevitable aspect of medical care and health care policy affecting the elderly. Furthermore, difficult ethical issues arise in the conduct of research on elderly subjects. However, to date, no federal resources have been allocated to conduct research on ethical issues concerning older persons. In order to carry out this important work, the federal government should apportion additional funds for research in biomedical ethics. An important step in this direction recently was taken by the National Institutes of Health's National Center for Human Genome Research, which earmarked 3 percent of its grant funds for study of ethical and social issues. Support for research on biomedical ethics in the treatment and study of older persons may help our society better understand and resolve these difficult dilemmas.

REFERENCES

American College of Physicians. 1989a. American College of Physicians ethics manual. Part 1: History; the patients; other physicians. Annals of Internal Medicine 111:245-252.
American College of Physicians. 1989b. American College of Physicians ethics manual, Part 2: Research, life-sustaining treatment; other issues. Annals of Internal Medicine 111:327-335.
Anderson, G. M., J. P. Newhouse, and L. L. Roos. 1989. Hospital care for elderly patients with diseases of the circulatory system: A comparison of hospital use in the United States and Canada. New England Journal of Medicine 321:1443-1448.
Annas, G. J. 1990. Nancy Cruzan and the right to die (Sounding Board). New England Journal of Medicine 323:670-672.
Annas, G. J., and L. H. Glantz. 1986a. The right of elderly patients to refuse life-sustaining treatment. Milbank Memorial Fund Quarterly; Health and Society 64(Supp. 2):95-162.
Annas, G. J., and L. H. Glantz. 1986b. Rules for research in nursing homes. New England Journal of Medicine 315:1157-1158.
Avorn, J. 1984. Benefit and cost analysis in geriatric care: Turning age discrimination into health policy. New England Journal of Medicine 310:955-959.
Bedell, S. E., and T. L. Delbanco. 1984. Choices about cardiopulmonary resuscitation in the hospital: When do physicians talk with patients? New England Journal of Medicine 310:1089-1093.
Brieger, G. 1978. Human experimentation history. Pp. 684-692 in The Encyclopedia of Bioethics, W. T. Reich, ed. New York: Free Press.
Brook, R. H. 1989. Practice guidelines and practicing medicine: Are they compatible? Journal of the American Medical Association 225:1159-1164.
Buchanan, A., and D. W. Brock. 1986. Deciding for others. Milbank Memorial Fund Quarterly; Health and Society 64(Supp. 2):17-94.
Callahan, D. 1987. Setting Limits: Medical Goals in an Aging Society. New York: Simon and Schuster.
Cassel, C. K. 1985. Research in nursing homes: Ethical issues. Journal of the American Geriatrics Society 33:795-799.
Cassel, C. K. 1987. Informed consent for research in geriatrics: History and concepts. Journal of the American Geriatrics Society 35:542-544.
Cassel, C. K. 1988. Ethical issues in the conduct of research in long-term care. Gerontologist 28(Supp.):90-96.
Cranford, R. E., and A. E. Doudera, eds. 1984. Institutional Ethics Committees and Health Care Decision Making. Ann Arbor, Mich.: Health Administration Press.
Daniels, N. 1986. Why saying no to patients in the United States is so hard. New England Journal of Medicine 314:1383-1386.
Dubler, N. 1987. Legal judgments and informed consent in geriatric research. Journal of the American Geriatrics Society 35:545-549.
Engelhardt, H. T., Jr., and M. A. Rie. 1986. Intensive care units, scarce resources, and conflicting principles of justice. Journal of the American Medical Association 225:1159-1164.
Faden, R. R., and T. L. Beauchamp. 1986. A History and Theory of Informed Consent. New York: Oxford University Press.
Fletcher, J. C., F. W. Dommel, and D. D. Cowell. 1985. Consent to research with impaired human subjects. Institutional Review Board 7:1-6.

Grumet, G. W. 1989. Health care rationing through inconvenience: The third party's secret weapon. New England Journal of Medicine 321:607-611.
Kane, N. M., and P. D. Manoukian. 1989. The effect of the Medicare prospective payment system on the adoption of new technology: The case of cochlear implants. New England Journal of Medicine 321:1378-1383.
Kane, R. A., and A. L. Caplan. 1989. Everyday Ethics: Resolving Dilemmas in Nursing Homes. New York: Springer Publishing.
Kapp, M., and B. Lo. 1986. Legal perceptions and their influence on medical decision making. Milbank Memorial Fund Quarterly; Health and Society 64(Supp.):163-202.
Leaf, A. 1989. Cost effectiveness as a criterion for Medicare coverage. New England Journal of Medicine 321:898-900.
Levine, R. J. 1986. Ethics and Regulation of Clinical Research. Baltimore, Md.: Urban and Schwarzenberg.
Lo, B. 1987. Behind closed doors: Promises and pitfalls of ethics committees. New England Journal of Medicine 317:46-49.
Lo, B. 1988. Quality of life judgments in the care of the elderly. Pp. 140-147 in Medical Ethics: A Guide for Health Care Professionals, D. C. Thomas and J. Monagle, eds. Rockville, Md.: Aspen Press.
Lo, B., and L. Dornbrand. 1986. The case of Claire Conroy: Will administrative review safeguard incompetent patients. Annals of Internal Medicine 104:869-873.
Lo, B., G. A. MacLeod, and G. Saika. 1986. Patient attitudes towards discussing life-sustaining treatment. Archives of Internal Medicine 146:1613-1615.
Lo, B., S. Rous, and L. Dornbrand. 1990. Family decision making on trial. Who decides for the patient? New England Journal of Medicine 322:1228-1232.
Miles, S. F., P. A. Singer, and M. Siegler. 1989. Conflicts between patients' wishes to forego treatment and the policies of health care facilities. New England Journal of Medicine 318:48-50.
Miller, F. H., and G. A. H. Miller. 1986. The painful prescription: A procrustean perspective? New England Journal of Medicine 314:1383-1386.
National Commission for the Protection of Human Subjects of Biomedical and Behavioral Research. 1978a. Report and Recommendations on Research Involving Those Institutionalized as Mentally Infirm. Washington, D.C.: U.S. Government Printing Office.
National Commission for the Protection of Human Subjects of Biomedical and Behavioral Research. 1978b. The Belmont Report: Ethical Principles and Guidelines for the Protection of Human Subjects of Research. Bethesda, Md: U.S. Government Printing Office.
President's Commission for the Study of Ethical Problems in Medicine and Biomedical and Behavioral Research. 1982. Making Health Care Decisions. Washington, D.C.: U.S. Government Printing Office.
President's Commission for the Study of Ethical Problems in Medicine and Biomedical and Behavioral Research. 1983. Deciding to Forgo Life-Sustaining Treatment. Washington, D.C.: U.S. Government Printing Office.
Ratzen, R. M. 1980. Being old makes you different: The ethics of research with elderly patients. Hastings Center Report 10:32-42.
Rhoden, N. K. 1988. Litigating life and death. Harvard Law Review 102:375-446.
Schneider, E. L. 1989. Options to control the rising health care costs of older Americans. Journal of the American Medical Association 261:907-908.
Scitovsky, A. A., and A. M. Capron. 1986. Medical care at the end of life: The

interaction of economics and ethics. Annual Review of Public Health 7:59-75.

Steinbrook, R., and B. Lo. 1988. Artificial feedings: Solid ground, not slippery slope. New England Journal of Medicine 318:286-290.

Tymchuck, A. J., J. G. Gouslander, B. Rahbar, and J. Fitten. 1988. Medical decision making among elderly people in long-term care. Gerontologist 28(Supp.):59-63.

Uhlmann, R. F., R. A. Pearlman, and K. C. Cain. 1988. Physicians' and spouses' predictions of elderly patients' resuscitation preferences. Journal of Gerontology 43: M115-M121.

Veatch, R. M. 1984. An ethical framework for terminal care decisions. Journal of the American Geriatrics Society 32:665-669.

Veatch, R. M. 1987. The Patient as Partner: A Theory of Human-Experimentation Ethics. Bloomington, Ind.: Indiana University Press.

Warren, J. W., J. Sobal, J. H. Tenney, J. M. Hoopes, D. Damron, S. Levenson, B. R. Deforge, and H. L. Muncie, Jr. 1986. Informed consent by proxy: An issue in research with elderly patients. New England Journal of Medicine 315:1125-1128.

Youngner, S. H. 1988. Who defines futility? Journal of the American Medical Association 260:2094-2095.

7
Review of Resources Committed to Research on Aging

It is difficult to identify the resources committed to research on aging. The limitations on measuring resources include the following: self-reporting by researchers; the absence of biologic markers to identify the research territory of old age; shared study targets, as in the examination of disorders found at several stages of life (e.g., diabetes, atherosclerosis, hypertension); the inclusion of administrative and training costs in research budgets; and the fact that basic discoveries in almost *any* area of biological science may contribute to the quality of life of older persons.

Despite these limitations, estimates of current support and future needs for research on aging are needed in order to promote realistic planning for this expanding area of study.

FUNDING SUPPORT FOR RESEARCH ON AGING

The Federal Government

National Institutes of Health

Most federal support comes from the National Institutes of Health (NIH). In fiscal year 1990, funds committed to the study of basic biomedical aspects of aging were about $442 million, or 5.8 percent of all NIH research funds, with $239 million coming from the National Institute on Aging (NIA) (Office of Planning, Technology,

Information and Evaluation, NIA). Table 7-1 summarizes funds for research on aging as reported by the institutes.

Department of Veterans Affairs

Veterans 65 and older constituted 27 percent of the veteran population in 1990, and this figure is expected to rise to 37 percent by the year 2000. The Department of Veterans Affairs (DVA) has been a leader in the development of research and training in geriatrics and gerontology in this country. In fiscal year 1990 the DVA reported about $17 million for age-related research, or 8.5 percent of the 1990 research budget of $201 million for the Department of Medicine and Surgery (Office of Assistant Chief Medical Director for Research and Development, DVA).

Alcohol, Drug Abuse, and Mental Health Administration

In fiscal year 1990 the Alcohol, Drug Abuse, and Mental Health Administration (ADAMHA) spent $42 million on research on aging, including $38 million on age-related research by the National Institute of Mental Health, or 4.9 percent of its total research budget of $855 million (Division of Financial Management, ADAMHA).

Health Care Financing Administration

The Health Care Financing Administration (HCFA) is the overseeing federal agency for Medicare and Medicaid, and in fiscal year 1990 it committed approximately $40 million to age-related studies, or about 82 percent of its research budget of $49 million for that year, largely in health services delivery (Office of Research and Demonstrations, HCFA). Most of this support was for demonstration projects; although demonstration projects can contribute to an understanding of aging, the committee believes that these funds cannot entirely be credited to support of research on aging.

Agency for Health Care Policy and Research

The Agency for Health Care Policy and Research (AHCPR) (formerly the National Center for Health Services Research and Health Care) spent $19 million on research on aging, or about 20 percent of its research budget of $95 million in fiscal year 1990 (Office of Financial Management, AHCPR). Most of the research supported was directed to the area of health services delivery.

TABLE 7-1 National Institutes of Health (NIH) Support for Research on Aging (in thousands of dollars)

Institute[a]	1989	1990	1991 (estimated)
National Institute on Aging (100)	$ 222,545	$ 238,927	$ 323,752
National Cancer Institute (1.1)	16,531	14,499	15,467
National Heart, Lung, and Blood Institute (2.1)	22,240	19,585	20,600
National Institute of Diabetes and Digestive Disorders (2.5)	14,127	20,800	21,700
National Institute of General Medical Sciences[b]			
National Institute of Neurological Disorders and Stroke (6.9)	33,141	35,920	45,975
National Institute of Allergy and Infectious Diseases (3.8)	28,506	32,998	35,678
National Eye Institute (13.4)	31,077	34,878	36,273
National Institute of Environmental Health Sciences (2.3)	1,696	1,917	1,997
National Institute of Arthritis and Musculo-skeletal and Skin Disorders (8.4)	13,590	13,995	15,744
National Institute of Deafness and Communicative Disorders (16.5)	1,511	7,947	9,007
National Center for Research Resources (2.8)	9,995	7,487	7,293
National Center for Nursing Research (11.3)	3,295	6,651	8,000
National Institute of Dental Research (4.2)	5,483	5,785	6,437
Office of Director (0.6)	461	400	400
Subtotal/aging	$ 404,198	$ 441,789	$ 548,323
(% of total budget)	(5.7%)	(5.8%)	(6.4%)
Total NIH budget	$7,152,207	$7,576,537	$8,511,782

[a]Numbers in parentheses are the percentage of the unit's 1989 budget allocated to research on aging.
[b]No support for research on aging identified.
SOURCE: Office of Planning, Technology, Information and Evaluation, NIA

Other Federal Departments and Agencies

Other agencies that provided support for research on aging included the Department of Agriculture, which committed $23 million in fiscal year 1990 for studies of nutrition in older persons (Office of Budget and Management Staff; Agriculture Research Service), and the Administration on Aging, which devoted about $3.0 million to research on aging that largely involved social and behavioral studies (Division of Research and Demonstrations) for the same year.

Industry and Foundations

Industry

Industry support for research on aging is difficult to measure because there is no central information repository. Indirect evidence comes from a review of the literature (see below), which showed that 5 percent of research papers on aging cited corporate support. A special case of research support by industry is that of the pharmaceutical companies. In 1989, U.S. companies spent more than $3.6 billion on research and development of drugs primarily used to treat diseases that afflict older patients (Pharmaceutical Manufacturers Association). This was 50 percent of the pharmaceutical industry's total research and development budget of $7.3 billion for the year. Cardiovascular disorders (stroke, heart disease, and hypertension) consumed 39 percent of the reported age-related research budget; the remainder of the budget supported investigation of drugs for the treatment of cancer, arthritis, and other conditions that afflict the geriatric population. Because most of these disorders also affect younger persons and because a significant portion of the funds went for development purposes, one cannot state with certainty how much of these funds actually supported age-related research.

Foundations

Information on foundation support for research on aging was obtained from the Foundation Center's 1989 publication *Grants for the Aged* and from a computer search of the center's on-line Grants Index. Both sources report information about corporate and foundation contributions of $5,000 or more. The Foundation Center reports that, from 1986 to early 1987, 2.5 percent of the monies given by private and corporate foundations were directed to the general area of aging, and less than 1 percent of all foundation philanthropy was for age-related research. In 1989, about $59 million was given for general projects in aging; of this sum, about $15 million (25 percent of all funds for projects in aging) went for studies specifically devoted to research on aging. The balance supported services, education, and administrative support for age-related programs. Foundations providing major support for research on aging included the Commonwealth Fund, New York; the Charles A. Dana Foundation, New York; the John A. Hartford Foundation, New York; the Henry J. Kaiser Family Foundation, California; the John D. and Catherine T. MacArthur Foundation, Illinois; the Robert Wood Johnson Foundation, New Jersey; the Weingart Foundation, California; and the Pew Charitable Trusts, Pennsylvania.

Information about state and local support of age-related research is difficult to obtain. A few states, such as California (through the statewide Academic Geriatric Research and Education Program) provide limited funds to support studies on aging. Local (city and county) support for research on aging could not be estimated because of the absence of any central source for such information.

INSTITUTIONS ENGAGED IN RESEARCH ON AGING

Centers for Research on Aging Supported by the NIA

Centers for the Study of Alzheimer's Disease

The NIA has established centers for basic science and clinical studies in Alzheimer's disease at the following institutions:

- Baylor College of Medicine, Texas
- Case Western Reserve University, Ohio
- Columbia University, New York
- Duke University, North Carolina
- Harvard University, Massachusetts
- Johns Hopkins University, Maryland
- Mount Sinai School of Medicine, New York
- University of California at San Diego
- University of Kentucky
- University of Michigan
- University of Pittsburgh, Pennsylvania
- University of Southern California
- University of Texas Southwestern Medical Center
- University of Washington
- Washington University (St. Louis), Missouri

Centers of Excellence in Research and Teaching in Geriatrics and Gerontology (Claude Pepper Centers)

Three Claude Pepper centers have been funded by the NIA. The NIA also provides funds for research in numerous university-based research centers through program project grants (P01). However, it is not always possible to characterize the centers receiving such funds as primarily age-oriented in their research activities.

Geriatric Research, Education, and Clinical Centers of the Department of Veterans Affairs

There are 7 million veterans 65 years old or older; half of all men in this country who are 65 and older are veterans. By the year 2000 there will be 9 million veterans 65 and over; 4 million of these will be 75 and over. In response to the needs of the veteran population the Geriatric Research, Education, and Clinical Centers (GRECC) program was initiated by act of Congress in 1975, and was expanded by further legislation in 1980. There are now 13 GRECCs, with 3 more planned for fiscal year 1991. Their purpose is to integrate basic research, teaching, and clinical achievements. Research activities of these centers are summarized in Table 7-2.

Teaching and Research Nursing Homes

The Robert Wood Johnson Foundation has sponsored eight teaching and research nursing homes affiliated with university medical schools. Research activities at these institutions are summarized in Table 7-3.

Other Institutional Supports for the Study of Aging

A noteworthy step by the private sector towards recruitment for careers in geriatrics took place in 1988, as the John A. Hartford Foundation initiated a strategy of supporting centers of excellence. The program, enhanced and broadened during 1989, encourages medical students and practicing physicians at 10 sites across the United States to specialize in academic geriatrics.

Although there are dozens of university centers for the study of aging across the country (including biomedical, behavioral and social, and health services delivery programs), a 1987 review of medical school-based fellowships in geriatrics identified only 13, at that time, as having an adequate complement of research and teaching personnel and implementing a full research program in aging (Institute of Medicine, 1987).

TABLE 7-2 DVA Geriatric Research, Education, and Clinical Centers

Location	Research Activities
Ann Arbor, Mich.	Neurosciences; metabolic and endocrine factors; autonomic function in diabetes mellitus and hypertension
Bedford, Mass.	Neurobiology of aging; immunology; rheumatology; computer-based clinical evaluation
Brockton-West Roxbury, Mass.	Influence of normal aging on homeostatic mechanisms: cardiovascular, endocrine, and neuroendocrine; carbohydrate metabolism
Durham, N.C.	Cancer and cardiovascular disease in aging; research on physical fitness
Gainesville, Fla.	Geropharmacology; molecular biology of aging; gene expression and aging; nutrition; neoplasms
Little Rock, Ark.	General basic and clinical research; role of antioxidants; motor and cognitive deficits
Minneapolis, Minn.	Study of Parkinson's disease; Alzheimer's disease
Palo Alto, Calif.	Endocrinology; metabolism; age-related changes in cognition; approaches to health delivery; depression
San Antonio, Tex.	Metabolism; endocrinology; nutrition; oral health and dentistry
Seattle, Wash.	Age-related changes in behavior and neuroendocrine function, and their relationship to health services
Sepulveda, Calif.	Endocrinology; memory; health services delivery
St. Louis, Mo.	General basic and clinical oncology; hypertension; gastroenterology; infectious disease; nephrology
West Los Angeles, Calif.	Basic science and clinical study of immunology; osteoporosis; evaluation of health care

SOURCE: DVA Department of Medicine and Surgery. Office of Geriatrics and Extended Care, Washington, D.C.

PUBLICATIONS ON RESEARCH IN AGING

The scientific literature represents an important resource for all future research activities. In order to estimate changes in the knowledge base and to identify trends in research activity in geriatrics and gerontology, the Institute for Scientific Information (ISI) undertook a screen of 500,000 articles from 1983 to 1987. Funding supports and

TABLE 7-3 Areas of Study at Teaching and Research Nursing Homes

Institution	Research Activities
University of California, San Diego	Nosocomial infections; predictors of institutionalization; sleep apnea
Yeshiva University	Dementia; osteoarthritis; motor control impairment; age-associated memory failure; congestive heart failure
Harvard University	Syncope and altered blood pressure; homeostasis in the elderly; urinary incontinence; vitamin D physiology and nutrition; risk of institutionalization; Alzheimer's disease: depression, neuroendocrine function
Case Western Reserve University	Respiratory and gastrointestinal infections; immune processes and tuberculosis; visual perception and Alzheimer's disease; neuroendocrine function in Alzheimer's disease
Johns Hopkins University	Metabolic regulation; cardiopulmonary physiology; sleep physiology; neuropsychological function
University of Pennsylvania	Urinary tract infection; regional cerebral structure and function in dementia; sleep apnea
Stanford University	Modifiable factors influencing health status/health care; hormones and hip fractures; cognitive function in diabetics; care in nursing homes
University of Iowa	Parkinson's disease; chronic conditions involving functional or cognitive impairment; interaction of stress and social supports

institutions of origin of scientific papers in 1982, 1983, and 1987 were assessed by ISI and by King Research, Inc., at the request of the Institute of Medicine.

In 1983, about 4,900 papers (or 1.7 percent of the total file of scientific reports) focused on aging; by 1987 the number of age-related research reports had risen to 8,900 (2.7 percent of the total file). The total file increased by 9 percent during this interval, resulting in an absolute increase in published studies on aging of 70 percent. Major areas of growth in the literature were in the neurosciences, including Alzheimer's disease, neurologic aging, cognition/memory, and Parkinson's disease. Reports in the area of neurological function and Alzheimer's disease increased fourfold. Second in growth were reports on infectious disease and osteoporosis in the aged. Social and psychological studies, health services delivery research, and pharmacology were well represented in both years, showing a modest increase in the number of publications between 1983 and 1987. Examination of the social and behavioral literature showed a high level of interest in geriatrics in 1983, but no striking change in the rate of publication was noted in the subsequent four years.

A further observation by the ISI review was that the increase in studies on aging involved many clearly defined areas of geriatric interest (e.g., studies of geriatric syndromes) with contributions made by many different fields of research (internal medicine, neurology, molecular biology, sociology, psychology). This observation demonstrates both the wide interest in the investigation of aging and the emergence of a body of information and research techniques that is focused on age-related topics.

Until recently, as the ISI findings indicated, aging studies not reported in publications clearly identified as focused on aging have tended to appear in professional journals devoted to behavioral and social science or to health services delivery research, with few reports appearing in medical and other scientific publications. That this trend has changed is illustrated, if not proven, by the increase between 1983 and 1987 in age-related studies reported in the selected medical and scientific journals shown in Table 7-4.

Although these peer-reviewed journals showed a more than 150 percent increase in publication of articles on research in aging between 1983 and 1987, further study is necessary to establish the presence of a significant trend. Of interest is the quadrupling of articles on aging in the neurology literature. During the period 1983 to 1987 there was also a significant increase in the number of journals devoted to the study of aging.

No support was listed for 16 percent of papers on age-related research in 1987; presumably, this support was provided by the institution of affiliation of the investigators. Among remaining papers, citations of support were divided as follows: government, 45 percent; foundations, 30 percent; foreign sources, 20 percent; and corporations, 5 percent.

PERSONNEL ENGAGED IN THE STUDY OF AGING

A 1980 study indicated that 7,000 to 10,300 geriatricians would be needed by the year 1990 (Kane et al., 1980). Based on staffing of 3 to 5 full-time faculty per teaching hospital and medical school, the

TABLE 7-4 Number of Age-Related Publications in Selected Journals

Journal	1983	1987
American Journal of Medicine	9	28
American Journal of Physiology	9	16
American Journal of Public Health	8	21
Annals of Internal Medicine	21	42
Annals of Neurology	17	54
Archives of Neurology	10	62
Brain Research	35	156
British Medical Journal	38	40
Journal of Clinical Investigation	5	9
Journal of Clinical Psychiatry	8	12
Journal of Comparative Neurology	20	72
Journal of Experimental Psychology	1	12
Journal of Neurochemistry	11	48
Journal of Neurology, Neuroscience and Psychiatry	12	41
Journal of Neuroscience	7	43
Journal of the American Medical Association	38	49
Lancet	36	56
Neurology	18	80
Neuropsychology	2	13
Neuroscience Letters	16	63
New England Journal of Medicine	31	65
Proceedings, National Academy of Sciences	9	40
Science	13	32
Social Science and Medicine	3	23
Total	377	1,077

SOURCE: Institute for Scientific Information, Philadelphia, Pa.

study predicted a need for 2,100 biomedical faculty to provide training for these geriatricians. It has been estimated that, by the year 2000, in order to meet the medical needs of the expanding older population, 10,000 to 21,000 geriatricians will be needed, and 14,000 to 29,000 will be needed by the year 2020 (NIA, 1988). Training of these physicians will require a major increase in staffing of departments of medicine and family practice by researchers and teachers with special competence in geriatrics and gerontology.

In 1987 the Institute of Medicine reported that only 100 geriatric fellows were graduating per year from hospital-based medical school programs. The report estimated that to meet requirements for an estimated 2,100 faculty by the year 2000 to train future clinicians and biomedical students of aging, the number of graduating fellows should be increased by at least 100 percent (Institute of Medicine, 1987). A report to Congress from the NIA (1988) and a study from the University of California at Los Angeles (Reuben, personal communication, 1990) support this recommendation. Although a recent report (Reuben et al., 1990) indicates that despite a recent upsurge in interest in geriatrics by internists and family practitioners, with as many as 5,000 certified geriatricians in practice by the mid-1990s, this is far short of the estimated minimum of 10,000 required by that time to provide adequate care of the older population.

A survey in 1986 of 400 graduates of geriatric biomedical fellowship programs showed that two-thirds held academic positions, but only 35 percent of those surveyed committed more than 10 percent of their time to teaching and research (Siu et al., 1989). The study pointed to a low rate of publication (1.3 papers per graduate annually) among the recent graduates compared with fellowship graduates in other disciplines, and it concluded that the goal of producing academic geriatricians is far from being met.

Thus, given even the most generous estimate of biomedical personnel engaged in research on aging, fewer than 150 graduates of fellowship programs in geriatrics spend more than 10 percent of their time in research. Balancing this estimate of the small number of researchers engaged in studies of aging is the observation that 15,047 authors were listed in geriatric and gerontological publications (including behavioral and health services research studies) in 1987, an increase of 34 percent over 1982 (King Research, Inc.). While this information cannot be interpreted as indicative of growth in the full-time complement of research investigators in aging, it points to a significant upward trend in the involvement of academic faculty in gerontologic and geriatric studies.

Biomedical age-related research is carried out by faculty M.D.s and biomedical Ph.D.s, with some studies in behavioral aspects of aging done by a small number of physician psychiatrists. The reports on training cited above did not measure the need for scientists and practitioners in behavioral or social studies, or in health services research. As noted in Chapters 4 and 5, support for training of Ph.D.s and other investigators in behavioral and social research or in health services delivery is inadequate, and the production of teachers and researchers in these fields must be expanded if *all* of the needs of the older generation are to be met. In a report to Congress (NIA, 1988) the NIA estimated the minimum requirements for faculty, including physicians, for the years 1990 and 2000 (Table 7-5). The estimates included faculty in the areas of psychology, pharmacology, and nursing, but did not include information about faculty to train social

TABLE 7-5 Faculty Needs in Age-Related Studies, 1990 and 2000

Faculty Work Place	1990	2000
Medical schools—physicians	600	1,300
Medical schools—other faculty	600	1,300
Nursing schools	750	1,500
Dental schools	80	120
Social work schools	300	1,000
Optometry schools	80	125
Pharmacy schools	150	300
Clinical psychology schools	150	450

SOURCE: National Institute on Aging (1988).

scientists or other nonbiomedical researchers on aging. The estimates, totaling about 2,900 faculty for the year 1990, and about 6,000 for the year 2000, were based on the expectation that 25 percent of physician time and 50 percent of the time of other faculty would be committed to research.

A 1987 report stated that the numbers of geriatric and gerontological faculty—including teachers and scientists in the fields of behavioral and social studies, and health services delivery—were inadequate to provide adequate training for health care personnel to meet the medical and nonmedical needs of older persons (NIA, 1988). In fiscal year 1990 the *total* number of trainees (biomedical; behavioral and social; neuroscience and neuropsychology) supported by the NIA was 425, a figure far short of the number required (Office of Planning, Technology, Information, and Evaluation, NIA).

The training of faculty must be increased sharply and as soon as possible if the recommended minimum goal of 6,000 additional faculty (biomedical and nonbiomedical) for research and teaching in age-related studies and the care of older persons is to be reached by the year 2000.

REFERENCES

Institute of Medicine. 1987. Academic geriatrics for the year 2000. Journal of the American Geriatrics Society 35:773-791.

Kane, R., D. Solomon, J. Beck, E. Keeler, and R. Kane. 1980. The future need for geriatric manpower in the United States. New England Journal of Medicine 302:1327-1332.

National Institute on Aging. 1988. Personnel for Health Needs of the Elderly Through the Year 2020. September 1987 Report to Congress. Document 1988-205-735-736:32533, U.S. Department of Health and Human Services. Washington, D.C.: U.S. Government Printing Office.

Reuben, D. B., T. B. Bradley, J. Zwanziger, J. H. Hirsh, and J. C. Beck. 1990. Candidates for the certificate of added qualifications in geriatric medicine. Who, why and when? Journal of the American Geriatrics Society 38:483-488.

Siu, A. L., G. Y. Ke, and J. C. Beck. 1989. Geriatric medicine in the United States. The current activities of former trainees. Journal of the American Geriatrics Society 37:272-276.

Appendixes

A

Acknowledgments

The Committee on a National Research Agenda on Aging and the Institute of Medicine are grateful for the contributions of the individuals listed below.

LIAISON TEAMS

Basic Biomedical Research

GEORGE M. MARTIN (Co-chair), Professor of Pathology, Adjunct Professor of Genetics, and Director, Alzheimer's Disease Research Center, University of Washington, Seattle

ROBERT T. SCHIMKE (Co-chair), American Cancer Society Research Professor of Biology, Stanford University, Stanford, California

PAUL BORNSTEIN, Professor of Biochemistry and Medicine, University of Washington, Seattle

CHARLES J. EPSTEIN Professor of Pediatrics and Biochemistry, School of Medicine, University of California, San Francisco

DONALD W. KING, Crane Professor of Pathology, Pritzker School of Medicine, Chicago, Illinois

CAROL B. LYNCH, Professor of Biology and Dean of the Sciences, Wesleyan University, Middletown, Connecticut

EDWARD J. MASORO, Professor and Chair, Department of Physiology, University of Texas Health Science Center, San Antonio
RICHARD A. MILLER, Associate Professor of Pathology and Biochemistry, Boston University School of Medicine, Boston, Massachusetts
CHARLES B. MOBBS, Assistant Professor of Neurobiology, Rockefeller University, New York, New York
PETER S. SPENCER, Professor of Neurology, and Director, Center for Research for Occupational and Environmental Toxicology, Oregon Health Sciences University, Portland
RICHARD L. SPROTT, Associate Director, Biomedical Research and Clinical Medicine, National Institute on Aging, Bethesda, Maryland
ROBERT E. STEVENSON, Director, American Type Culture Collection, Rockville, Maryland
DAVID WARD, Professor of Human Genetics, Molecular Biophysics, and Biochemistry, Yale University Medical School, New Haven, Connecticut

Clinical Research

WILLIAM APPLEGATE (Co-chair), Chief, Division of Geriatric Medicine, and Professor of Preventive Medicine, University of Tennessee, Memphis
WILLIAM HAZZARD (Co-chair), Professor and Chair, Department of Internal Medicine, Bowman Gray School of Medicine, Wake Forest University, Winston-Salem, North Carolina
WILLIAM ADLER, Chief, Clinical Immunology Section, National Institute on Aging, Baltimore, Maryland
BRUCE J. BAUM, Clinic Director and Chief, Clinical Investigations and Patient Care Branch, National Institute of Dental Research, Bethesda, Maryland
EVAN CALKINS, Professor of Medicine, State University of New York at Buffalo
LARRY G. DUCKERT, Associate Professor, Department of Otolaryngology, University of Washington School of Medicine, Seattle
WALTER ETTINGER, Associate Professor of Internal Medicine and Chief, Section on Internal Medicine and Gerontology, Bowman Gray School of Medicine, Wake Forest University, Winston-Salem, North Carolina

ANDREW GOLDBERG, Associate Professor of Medicine, Johns Hopkins School of Medicine, Baltimore, Maryland
JAMES G. GOODWIN, Professor and Vice Chair, Department of Medicine, Medical College of Wisconsin, Milwaukee
EVAN C. HADLEY, Chief, Geriatrics Branch, National Institute on Aging, Bethesda, Maryland
JEFFREY B. HALTER, Professor of Internal Medicine and Chair, Division of Geriatric Medicine, University of Michigan Medical School, Ann Arbor
DAVID HAMERMAN, Professor of Medicine, Division of Geriatrics, Albert Einstein School of Medicine, Bronx, New York
ROBERT KATZMAN, Professor and Chair, Department of Neurosciences, University of California, San Diego, School of Medicine, La Jolla
ZAVEN KHACHATURIAN, Associate Director for Neuroscience and Neuropsychology of Aging, National Institutes of Health, Bethesda, Maryland
EDWARD G. LAKATTA, Head, Laboratory of Cardiovascular Science, Gerontology Research Center, National Institute on Aging, Baltimore, Maryland
PHILLIP LANDFIELD, Professor of Physiology, Bowman Gray School of Medicine, Winston-Salem, North Carolina
LEWIS A. LIPSITZ, Assistant Professor of Medicine, Harvard Medical School, Boston, Massachusetts
KENNETH W. LYLES, Assistant Professor of Medicine, Duke University Medical Center, Durham, North Carolina
MAURICE B. MITTELMARK, Associate Professor of Public Health Science, Bowman Gray School of Medicine, Wake Forest University, Winston-Salem, North Carolina
ELLIOT RAPAPORT, Professor of Medicine, School of Medicine, University of California, San Francisco
BURTON V. REIFLER, Professor and Chair, Department of Psychiatry and Behavioral Medicine, Bowman Gray School of Medicine, Wake Forest University, Winston-Salem, North Carolina
NEIL M. RESNICK, Associate Professor of Medicine, Harvard Medical School, Boston, Massachusetts
JAMES E. TURNER, Professor of Anatomy and Associate in Ophthalmology, Bowman Gray School of Medicine, Winston-Salem, North Carolina
MARK WILLIAMS, Associate Professor of Medicine, School of Medicine, University of North Carolina, Chapel Hill

THOMAS YOSHIKAWA, Assistant Chief Medical Director, Extended Care, Department of Veterans Affairs, Washington, D.C.

Behavioral and Social Sciences

Behavioral Sciences

LEONARD W. POON (Co-chair), Professor of Psychology and Director, Gerontology Center, University of Georgia, Athens

JAMES S. JACKSON, Professor of Psychology, University of Michigan, Ann Arbor

ALFRED KASZNIAK, Professor of Psychology, University of Arizona, Tucson

WARNER SCHAIE, Professor and Director, Gerontology Center, Human Development Department of Individual and Family Studies, Pennsylvania State University, University Park

ILENE SIEGLER, Associate Professor, Medical Psychology and Psychiatry, Duke University Medical Center, Durham, North Carolina

HARVEY STERNS, Professor and Director, Institute for Life Span Development and Gerontology, University of Akron, Akron, Ohio

DIANA WOODRUFF-PAK, Professor of Psychology, Temple University, Philadelphia, Pennsylvania

STEVE ZARIT, Professor and Assistant Director, Gerontology Center, Human Development Department of Individual and Family Studies, Pennsylvania State University, University Park

Social Sciences

GEORGE L. MADDOX (Co-chair), University Council on Aging and Human Development, Duke University, Durham, North Carolina

VERN L. BENGTSON, Director, Gerontology Research Institute, University of Southern California, Los Angeles

DAN G. BLAZER, Professor of Psychiatry, Duke University Medical Center, Durham, North Carolina

RICHARD CAMPBELL, Department of Sociology, University of Illinois at Chicago, Chicago, Illinois

ROBERT L. CLARK, Department of Economics and Business, North Carolina State University, Raleigh

JENNIE KEITH, Department of Sociology and Anthropology, Swarthmore College, Swarthmore, Pennsylvania

JILL QUADAGNO, Institute on Aging, Florida State University, Tallahassee

Health Services Delivery Research

MERWYN R. GREENLICK (Chair), Vice President (Research) and Director, Center for Health Research, Kaiser Permanente, Northwest Region; and Professor and Acting Chair, Department of Public Health and Preventive Medicine, Oregon Health Sciences University, Portland

PATRICIA ARCHBOLD, Professor, Department of Family Nursing, School of Nursing, Oregon Health Sciences University, Portland

DALE B. CHRISTIANSEN, Department of Pharmacy Practice, School of Pharmacy, University of Washington, Seattle

MARK HORNBROOK, Senior Investigator, Kaiser Permanente, Center for Health Research, Portland, Oregon

GLENN HUGHES, Director, Geriatric Education Center, and Co-director, Center of Aging, University of Alabama, Birmingham

RICHARD E. JOHNSON, Senior Investigator, Kaiser Permanente Center for Health Research, Portland, Oregon

DAVID A. KNAPP, Chair, Pharmacy Practices and Administrative Sciences, School of Pharmacy, University of Maryland, Baltimore

WALTER LEUTZ, Associate Research Professor, Brandeis University, Waltham, Massachusetts

BENTSON MCFARLAND, Assistant Professor of Psychiatry, Oregon Health Sciences University, Portland, Oregon

CHARLOTTE MULLER, Professor, Economics and Sociology, City University of New York, New York

SAM SHAPIRO, Professor Emeritus, Health Policy and Management, Johns Hopkins University, Baltimore, Maryland

Biomedical Ethics

CHRISTINE CASSELL, Professor of Medicine, University of Chicago School of Medicine, Chicago, Illinois

BERNARD LO, Associate Professor of Medicine and Director, Program in Medical Ethics, University of California School of Medicine, San Francisco

EXPERTS PROVIDING INFORMATION TO THE COMMITTEE

ROBERT BERG, Professor and Chair, Department of Preventive, Family, and Rehabilitative Medicine, Strong Memorial Hospital, Rochester, New York

BRIAN BILES, Staff Director, Subcommittee on Health, Committee on Ways and Means, U.S. House of Representatives, Washington, D.C.

DAVID M. BOROFSKI, American College of Physicians, Philadelphia, Pennyslvania

GENE COHEN, Deputy Director, National Institute on Aging, Bethesda, Maryland

SHARON L. COHEN, Director, Health Policy, Alliance for Aging Research, Washington, D.C.

KATHLEEN GARDNER CRAVEDI, Staff Director, Select Committee on Aging, U.S. House of Representatives, Washington, D.C.

STEVE CUMMINGS, Assistant Professor, School of Medicine, University of California, San Francisco

MARY C. CUSHING, Chief, Extramural Financial Data Branch, National Cancer Institute, Bethesda, Maryland

ANN J. DAVIS, Professor, Mental Health, Community, and Administrative Nursing, School of Medicine, University of California, San Francisco

ROBERT H. EBERT, Chair, Grants Monitoring Program, The Commonwealth Fund, New York, New York

HAROLD EPSTEIN, Executive Director, American Federation for Aging Research, New York, New York

CAROL GOODWIN, Associate Executive Vice President, American Geriatrics Society, New York, New York

BARBARA R. GREENBERG, Executive Director, Florence V. Burden Foundation, New York, New York

MARY S. HARPER, Coordinator, Long-Term Care Programs, National Institute of Mental Health, Rockville, Maryland

DeWITT G. HAZZARD, Head, Office of Resource Development, Biomedical Research and Clinical Medicine Program, National Institute on Aging, Bethesda, Maryland

JANE HEIDT, Indegate, Incorporated, New York, New York

LINDA HIDDEMAN BARONDESS, Executive Vice President, American Geriatrics Society, New York, New York

MO KATZ, Senior Program Advisor, The Commonwealth Fund, New York, New York

THOMAS KICKHAM, Deputy Director, Office of Research and

APPENDIX A

Demonstrations, Health Care Financing Administration, Baltimore, Maryland
SAM KORPER, Assistant Director, National Institute on Aging, Bethesda, Maryland
PHILLIP R. LEE, Director, Institute for Health Policy Studies, University of California, San Francisco
JAMES J. LEONARD, Chair, Department of Medicine, Uniformed Services University of the Health Sciences, Bethesda, Maryland
DONALD LINDBERG, Director, National Library of Medicine, Bethesda, Maryland
ADRIENNE A. LINDGREN, Grants Manager, The Commonwealth Fund, New York, New York
JANE MALLOY, Deputy Director for Policy, U. S. Department of Commerce, Washington, D.C.
PAUL A. MARKS, President and Chief Executive Officer, Memorial Sloan Kettering Cancer Center, New York, New York
MANUEL MIRANDA, Staff Director, Select Committee on Aging, U.S. House of Representatives, Washington, D.C.
PORTIA MITTELMAN, Staff Director, U.S. Senate Special Committee on Aging, Washington, D.C.
ROBERT F. MOORE, Head, Special Projects and Presentations, Statistical and Evaluation Unit, Division of Research Grants, National Institutes of Health, Bethesda, Maryland
MATTHEW A. MOVSESIAN, Assistant Professor of Medicine, University of Utah School of Medicine, Salt Lake City
GILBERT S. OMENN, Dean, School of Public Health, University of Washington, Seattle
DAN PERRY, Executive Director, Alliance for Aging Research, Washington, D.C.
EVA RAY, Steg, Ray and Associates, Villanova, Pennsylvania
DONNA REGENSTREIF, Senior Program Officer, The John A. Hartford Foundation, New York, New York
DAVID REUBEN, Associate Director, Multicampus Division, Geriatrics, University of California, School of Medicine, Los Angeles
REBECCA RIMEL, Executive Director, The Pew Charitable Trusts, Philadelphia, Pennsylvania
JOAN ROSENBACH, Program Analyst, Department of Health and Human Services, Washington, D.C.
KAREN S. ROSS, Chief, Financial Management and Information

Systems Branch, National Institute on Aging, Bethesda, Maryland
DAVID B. RUBIN, Associate Director, Multicampus Division of Geriatric Medicine and Gerontology, University of California, Los Angeles
CHARLES L. SCHEPENS, President, Eye Research Institute, Boston, Massachusetts
ROSEANNE SIEGEL, Program Officer, The Pew Charitable Trusts, Philadelphia, Pennsylvania
STANLEY L. SLATER, Director, Geriatric Research and Training Program, Geriatrics Branch, Biomedical Research and Clinical Training Medicine Program, National Institute on Aging, Bethesda, Maryland
JANE TAKEUCHI, Senior Research Associate, American Association of Retired People, Washington, D.C.
LILLIAN TROLL, Adjunct Professor, School of Medicine, University of California, San Francisco
JOAN VAN NOSTRAND, Deputy Director, Division of Health Care Statistics, Hyattsville, Maryland
JAMES D. WATSON, Director, National Center for Human Genome Research, National Institutes of Health, Bethesda, Maryland
MYRON WEISFELDT, Director, Clayton Heart Center, Johns Hopkins Hospital, Baltimore, Maryland
MARINA WEISS, Staff Director, Committee on Finance, U.S. Senate, Washington, D.C.
MARTIN WENGLENSKY, Professor of Sociology, Quinnipiac College, Hamden, Connecticut
CYNTHIA WOODCOCK, Assistant Vice President, The Commonwealth Fund, New York, New York
JAMES B. WYNGAARDEN, Foreign Secretary, National Academy of Sciences, Washington, D.C.

DIRECTORS, DVA GERIATRIC RESEARCH, EDUCATION, AND CLINICAL CENTERS

HARVEY J. COHEN, Department of Veterans Affairs Medical Center, Durham, North Carolina
BERNARD B. DAVIS, Department of Veterans Affairs Medical Center, St. Louis, Missouri
DAVID A. LIPSCHITZ, Department of Veterans Affairs Medical Center, Little Rock, Arkansas

TAKASHI MAKINODAN, Department of Veterans Affairs Medical Center, West Los Angeles, California
JOHN E. MORLEY, Department of Veterans Affairs Medical Center, Sepulveda, California

DIRECTORS, PHARMACEUTICAL COMPANY RESEARCH

WILLIAM ABRAMS, Executive Director, Scientific Development, Merck, Sharpe, and Dohme, Rahway, New Jersey
LIONEL EDWARDS, Director, Clinical Research, Schering-Plough, Kenilworth, New Jersey
ELKAN GAMZU, Senior Director, Drug Development, Parke Davis, Ann Arbor, Michigan
JAMES GAYLOR, Director, Molecular Biology, Johnson and Johnson Company, New Brunswick, New Jersey
JOHN GODFREY, Associate Director, Clinical Research, Rorer Central Research, Horsham, Pennsylvania
ROBERT LEWIS, Director, Basic Research, Syntex Corporation, Palo Alto, California
ERIC MUTH, Director, Central Nervous System Clinical Research, Wyeth Ayerst Research, Monmouth, New Jersey
RAJESH SHROTRIYA, Director, Central Nervous System Clinical Research, Bristol Myers Company, Wallingford, Connecticut
W. LEIGH THOMPSON, Group Vice President, Eli Lilly and Company, Indianapolis, Indiana
MICHAEL TIDD, Director, Medical Division, Norwich-Eaton Pharmaceuticals, Inc., Norwich, New York

B

Background Documents

For this study, the Institute of Medicine invited reports on various topics concerning research in aging. The manuscripts of four of these documents are available from the National Technical Information Service, 5285 Port Royal Road, Springfield, VA 22161, (703) 487-4650.

- "Opportunities in Basic Biomedical Research," Basic Biomedical Research Liaison Team, Institute of Medicine.
- "Opportunities in Clinical Research," Clinical Research Liaison Team, Institute of Medicine.
- "Opportunities in Behavioral and Social Sciences Research," Behavioral and Social Sciences Liaison Team, Institute of Medicine.
- "Opportunities in Health Services Delivery Research," Health Services Delivery Research Liaison Team, Institute of Medicine.

Index

A

Academic research, 4-5, 124, 129-130
Activities of daily living, 58-59
Agency for Health Care Policy and Research, 23, 120
Aging, Our Future Selves, 2, 3
Aging process, general, 2, 3, 44, 45, 48, 49
    brain, 10
    defined, 9, 47
    differential, 17, 51, 71, 72, 73-74, 77
    diseases and, 9-10, 14-16, 42, 44, 47-48, 62-66
    multidisciplinary approach, 9, 49
    nutrition and, 16
    productivity, 77, 79, 80, 82
    senescence, general, 9, 10, 11, 47, 51, 54-55, 65
    social-psychological, 17-20, 71, 75-77, 78-80
Alcohol, Drug Abuse, and Mental Health Administration, 20, 103, 120
Alzheimer's disease, 5, 6-7, 14, 41, 50, 53, 63-64, 99, 126
    genetics, 10, 11, 49, 51, 64, 68
Alzheimer's Disease Research Centers, 54, 123

Animal research, 11, 33, 34, 48, 51, 53
    ethics, 24
Atherosclerosis, 10, 14, 49, 54, 63, 66
Attitudes
    professionals, 94
    research participants, 114

B

Behavioral sciences, 2, 3, 16, 25, 71-75, 127, 138
    brain, 84-85
    clinical studies, relations to, 18, 24-25
    databases, 78, 83
    differential aging, 17, 51, 71, 72, 73-74, 77
    funding, 20, 30, 82-83
    lifestyle risk factors, 55, 59, 100
    longitudinal studies, 17, 19, 71, 81, 82, 83
    multidisciplinary approach, 25, 46, 58, 71, 72, 73, 81-82, 83-85
    neurobehavioral approach, 18, 73, 76
    research, priority, 17-19, 75-80
    research, secondary, 20, 81

145

technological innovations, effects, 19, 80, 94
urinary incontinence, 14
see also Health promotion; Mental health and illness; Psychology and psychiatry; Social sciences and services
Biomedical ethics, 3, 23, 46, 107, 139
  animal research, 24
  clinical research, 23, 25, 68–69, 113–115
  competency issues, 23, 108, 109, 114
  drugs, 69
  funding, 107, 115
  genetics, 24
  informed consent, 23, 69, 108, 109, 113–114
  institutionalized persons, 23, 108, 110
  life-sustaining treatments, 23, 108–110
  long-term care, 23, 108, 110, 114–115
  Medicare, 111
  nursing homes, 109, 110, 114–115
  research, priority, 23, 107–115
  research, secondary, 23–24, 115
  resource allocation, 23, 24, 95, 111–113
Biomedical research, basic, 9–10, 46, 47–55, 135–136
  funding, 11–12, 30, 50–55
  longitudinal studies, 11–12, 53–55
  multidisciplinary approach, 24, 55, 58
  professional education, 12, 24, 54
  research, priority, 10, 49–50
  research, secondary, 10–11, 50–52
  see also specific subdisciplines
Bone diseases, *see* Musculoskeletal system
Brain, 10, 18, 73, 84–85
  see also Cognitive abilities
Brookdale Foundation, 36

C

Cancer, 15, 49, 54, 65–66, 68
  cellular carcinogenesis, 10
Cardiovascular system, 6, 14, 59, 63, 77–78, 110
  atherosclerosis, 10, 14, 49, 54, 63, 66
  cellular studies, general, 11, 50
  hypertension, 14, 25, 59, 63, 66, 76

Case management, 22
Cell biology, 48, 50, 52, 53
  cardiovascular system, 11, 50
  dementia, 15, 64, 68
  genetics, 11, 55, 63
  homeostasis, 10, 16, 49, 54–55, 66
  neurons, 11, 50
  postmitotic, 11, 50
Centers of Excellence in Geriatric and Gerontological Research and Training, 12, 16, 32–33, 54, 67, 83, 102, 124
Chronic diseases, 2, 6–7, 41, 91
  life expectancy and, 8, 77–78
  mental, 20, 81; *see also* Dementia
  see also Disabilities; Long-term care; *specific diseases*
Claude Pepper Centers, *see* Centers of Excellence in Geriatric and Gerontological Research and Training
Clinical science, 2, 3, 24–25, 57–58, 136–138
  behavioral, 18, 24–25
  databases, 12, 57
  dementia, 59, 63–64
  disabilities, 12–13, 57, 58–62, 68
  ethical issues, 23, 25, 68–69, 113–115
  funding, 16, 67–68
  genetics, 24–25
  multidisciplinary approach, 24–25, 57–58, 68–69
  professional education 16, 67–68
  research, priority, 12–16, 58–66
  research, secondary, 16, 66–67
  see also Health promotion; Health services delivery; Pharmacological agents; Rehabilitation
Cognitive abilities, 18, 77
  delirium, 14, 62
  learning, 17, 18, 75, 77
  memory, 18, 75, 76, 77, 84–85
  see also Dementia
Commonwealth Fund, vii, 123
Competency issues, 23, 108, 109
  see also Informed consent
Computers and computer science, 22
  databases, 11–12, 34, 45, 57, 78, 83, 96, 97
Consent, *see* Informed consent
Construction of facilities, 26, 34–35
Cost factors
  clinical research, 58
  construction, 26, 34–35
  disabled, care of, 1–2, 8, 21, 111
  drugs, 96, 98

INDEX

employer cost sharing, 22, 102
geriatric syndromes, 61, 62
infrastructure, 33–34
long-term care, 21, 101, 111
Medicare, 7, 111, 120
musculoskeletal disorders, 15, 64
overall, 7, 20, 89, 95–96, 101, 111
professional education, 32
reduction of, 3, 8, 58
research, priority, 101
urinary incontinence, 14
Criteria for selection of priorities, 3, 44
Crosscutting issues, 24–25, 55, 68–69, 83–86, 103–104
Cultural factors, 17, 25, 45, 53, 72–73, 77–78, 84

D

Charles A. Dana Foundation, 123
Databases, 34, 45, 96
 archival, 11–12
 behavioral research, 78, 83
 clinical research, 12, 57
 pharmacological, 97
Decision making
 life-sustaining treatments, 23, 108–110
 resource allocation, ethical issues, 23, 24, 95, 111–113
 surrogate, 108, 109, 114
 see Competency issues; Informed consent
Delirium, 14, 62
Dementia, 1, 6–7, 14–15, 20, 99, 126
 cellular studies, 15, 64, 68
 clinical research, 59, 63–64
 see also Alzheimer's disease
Demographic factors, 1, 45, 77–78, 81–82, 84, 88, 100, 103
 drug expenditures, 98
 epidemiology, 53, 77–78, 81–82, 103
 funding of research, 30–31, 34
 gender differences, 25, 45, 53, 55, 68, 74, 78, 83–84, 103
 morbidity and mortality, 3, 6, 7–8, 18–19, 77–78, 81
 poverty, 2, 18, 74, 78, 93, 95, 113
 race/ethnicity, 17, 25, 45, 53, 68, 72, 74, 78, 79, 84, 95, 103
 socioeconomic status, general, 78, 79, 84, 95, 103
Demonstration projects, 92–93, 97, 100, 120
Dental and oral diseases, 16, 66

Department of Health and Human Services
 education and training, 32
 see also National Institutes of Health; other specific agencies
Department of Veterans Affairs, 120, 124, 125, 142–143
 research and training, 5, 6
Dependence/independence, 2, 6, 7–8, 90, 91
 activities of daily living, 58–59
 behavioral interventions, 16–17, 81
 drug management, 61
 employment, 19
 functional capacity, 44
Diabetes, 6, 16, 53
Diet, see Nutrition
Differential aging, 17, 51, 71, 72, 73–74, 77
Disabilities, 3, 6–7, 41, 49, 89
 behavioral studies, 18–19
 clinical studies, 12–13, 57, 58–62, 68
 cost of care, 1–2, 8, 21, 111
 defined, 6
 disease and, 100
 health promotion, 22, 100
 life expectancy and, 8
 musculoskeletal system, 13
 reductions in, 2
 see also Long-term care; Rehabilitation; specific disabling diseases
Diseases and disorders, 3
 aging process and, general, 9–10, 14–16, 42, 44, 62–63
 disability and, 100
 psychological concomitants, 20
 senescence, general, 9, 10, 11, 47, 51, 54–55, 65
 see also Chronic diseases; Infectious diseases; Morbidity and mortality; specific diseases and anatomical systems
Drugs, see Pharmacological agents

E

Economic factors, 74
 see also Cost factors; Financial factors; Poverty; Socioeconomic status
Education, 74
 see also Professional education
Employment and unemployment, 19, 78, 93, 96
 cost sharing by employer, 22, 102

geriatrics personnel, 127–130
long-term care workers, 93, 96
productivity and aging, 77, 79, 80, 82
retirement, 19, 76–77, 79, 82
women, 89, 93
Endocrinology, 11, 50, 76
Environmental factors, 9, 11, 18, 45, 51, 52, 66, 72–73, 74
see also Cultural factors; Nutrition; Social sciences; Technological innovation
Epidemiology, 53, 77–78, 81–82, 103
Ethics, see Biomedical ethics
Ethnicity; see Cultural factors; Race/ethnicity

F

Failure to thrive, 13, 60
Families, 23, 110–111
decisions about elderly, surrogate, 108, 109, 114
long-term care, 90, 91–92, 93–94, 96
social support structures, 79
Federal government, general see Funding; Regulations; Standards; specific departments and agencies
Field studies, 72, 82
Financial factors, 89, 95–96, 101, 119–123
long-term care, 21, 82, 90
see also Cost factors; Funding
Foundations, 26, 35–36, 37, 82, 103, 122–123
Funding, 2, 26–37, 45, 119–130
allocation, ethical issues, 23, 24, 95, 111–113
behavioral sciences, 20, 30, 82–83
biomedical research, basic, 11–12, 30, 50–55
clinical research, 16, 67–68
demography, 30–31, 34
ethics research, 107, 115
health promotion, 30–31
health services delivery, 22–23, 102–103, 112–113

G

Gender differences, 25, 45, 53, 55, 68, 74, 78, 83–84, 103
see also Women

Genetics, 9–10, 11, 15, 46, 47–48, 50, 51–52, 63
Alzheimer's disease, 10, 11, 49, 51, 64, 68
cancer, 15, 65–66
cardiovascular diseases, 14
cellular, 11, 55, 63
clinical studies, relations to, 24–25
ethics research, 24
immune system, 65
metabolism and homeostasis, 16, 66
methodology, 48–49
musculoskeletal disorders, 15, 16, 65
nutrition and, 63, 66
Geriatric Research and Training Centers, see Centers of Excellence in Geriatric and Gerontological Research and Training
Geriatrics and gerontology, 2, 42, 49
personnel, 127–130
syndromes, 12, 13–14, 57, 60–62
see also Professional education
Government role, see Funding; Regulations; Standards; specific departments and agencies
Grants, see Funding

H

Handicaps, see Disabilities
John A. Hartford Foundation, 123, 124
Health Care Financing Administration, 20, 23, 30, 83, 90, 120
Medicare, 7, 96, 111, 120
Health promotion, 18, 21, 45–46, 49, 59, 62, 63, 74–75, 89, 100
disabilities, 22, 100
during chronic illness, 20
field studies, 72, 82
funding, 30–31
Medicare, 96
research, priority, 13, 22, 101, 102
resource allocation, ethical issues, 112
Health services delivery, 3, 20–21, 25, 46, 88–100, 139
case management, 22
costs, 1–2, 8, 21, 111
equity and access, 111–113
funding, 22–23, 102–103, 112–113
mental health, 22, 89, 99–100
multidisciplinary approach, 22, 25, 58, 103–104

professional education, 88–89, 93, 103
research, priority, 21–22, 89, 101–102
research, secondary, 22, 102
research vs, care, 112–113
see also Institutionalized persons; Long-term care; Nursing homes
Heart disease, see Cardiovascular system
Home care, 90, 91–92, 93–94, 96
  costs, 8
Homeostasis, 10, 16, 49, 54–55, 66
Hypertension, 14, 25, 59, 63, 66, 68, 76

I

Imaging, 15
Immune system, 49, 50–51, 65
  infectious diseases, 15, 65, 127
  vaccines, 15, 65
Independence, see Dependence/independence
Infectious diseases, 15, 65, 127
Information
  databases, 11–12, 34, 45, 57, 78, 83, 96, 97
  publications, 40–41, 43, 125–127, 128, 129
  see also specific publications
Informed consent, 23, 69, 108, 113–114
  surrogate, 108, 109, 114
Infrastructure, 22, 33–34, 50, 68
  computers and computer science, 22
  construction costs, 26, 34–35
  databases, 11–12, 34, 45, 57, 78, 83, 96, 97
  laboratories, 33, 54
  see also Centers of Excellence in Geriatric and Gerontological Research and Training; Computers and computer science
Institute for Scientific Information, 125–127
Institute of Medicine, 2, 4, 37, 42, 58, 67
Institutionalized persons, 22, 75, 92–93, 102
  demented, 64
  ethical issues, 23, 108, 110
Instrumental activities of daily living, see Activities of daily living
Interdisciplinary approach, see Multidisciplinary approach

J

Robert Wood Johnson Foundation, 123, 124

K

Henry J. Kaiser Family Foundation, 123

L

Laboratories, 33, 54
  construction of, 26, 34–35
  see also Centers of Excellence in Geriatric and Gerontological Research and Training
Learning, 17, 18, 75, 77
Legal issues
  litigation, 110
  mandatory retirement, 19, 76, 79–80
  see also Competency issues; Informed consent; Regulations
Life expectancy, 6, 7, 11, 45–46
  behavioral/social factors, 74
  chronic illness and, 8, 77–78
  gender differences, 78
  methodological issues, 51
  nutrition, 51
Litigation, 110
Longitudinal studies, 34, 45, 103–104
  behavioral/social, 17, 19, 71, 81, 82, 83
  biomedical research, basic, 11–12, 53–55
  clinical research, 13
  gender differences, 78
Long-term care, 57, 89, 90–94, 95
  behavioral interventions, 81
  costs, 21, 101, 111
  defined, 90
  ethical issues, research, 23, 108, 110, 114–115
  family providers, 90, 91–92, 93–94, 96
  financing, 21, 82, 90
  institutionalized persons, 22, 23, 64, 75, 92–93, 102, 108, 110
  methodology, 92–93
  models, 102
  nursing homes, 7, 8, 14, 93–94, 99, 109, 110, 114–115, 124, 126
  personnel, 93, 96
  quality of life, 91, 92, 94

rehabilitation, 13, 57, 58–59, 76, 111
research, priority, 21, 101

M

John D. and Catherine T. MacArthur Foundation, 123
Medicare, 120
   costs, 7, 111, 120
   data about, 96
   ethical issues, 111
Medications, see Pharmacological agents
Memory, 18, 75, 76, 77, 84–85
Mental health and illness, 21
   chronic illness, 20, 81
   delirium, 14, 62
   research, priority, 22, 101, 102
   research, secondary, 89
   services delivery, 22, 89, 99–100
   see also Cognitive abilities; Dementia; Psychology and psychiatry
Metabolic disorders, 16, 66
Methodology
   behavioral/social, 81–82
   biomedical, basic, 9–10
   field studies, 72, 82
   long-term care research, 92–93
   molecular biology and genetics, 48–49
   of present study, 2–4, 42–44
   senescence research, 51
   see also Longitudinal studies; Multidisciplinary approach
Minorities, see Race/ethnicity
Mobility, 13, 60–61
Models, 52
   aging and lifespan, 11
   animal, 11, 24, 33, 34, 48, 51, 53
   behavioral/social research, 81
   long-term care, 102
   reproductive system as, 51
Molecular genetics, see Genetics
Morbidity and mortality, 3, 6, 7–8, 18–19, 68, 77–78
   databases, 11–12, 78, 96
   demography and, 3, 6, 7–8, 18–19, 77–78, 81
   drug mismanagement, 61
   epidemiology, 53, 77–78, 81–82, 103
   funding, 30–31
   geriatric syndromes, 61, 62, 63
   postponed morbidity, 18–19, 75, 77–78

senescence, general, 9, 10, 11, 47, 51, 54–55, 65
   see also Disabilities; Life expectancy
Multidisciplinary approach, 4, 24–25, 44–45, 48
   aging process, 9, 49
   behavioral/social research, 25, 46, 58, 71, 72, 73, 81–82, 83–85
   biomedical, basic, 24, 55, 58
   clinical research, 24–25, 57–58, 68–69
   construction of centers, 22, 34
   dementia, 15
   drug management, 61, 97
   health services delivery, 22, 25, 58, 103–104
   professional education, 24, 55
   quality of life index, 19–20, 80–81
   see also Centers of Excellence in Geriatric and Gerontological Research and Training
Musculoskeletal system, 13, 15, 16, 50, 60–61, 64–65, 66
   disease costs, 15, 64
   genetics, 15, 16, 65
   osteoarthritis, 10, 15, 49, 54, 64
   osteoporosis, 8, 15, 59, 64, 64, 127

N

National Center for Human Genome Research, 24
National Health Interview Survey, 58
National Institute of Aging, 5, 11–12, 28–30, 35, 43, 119–120, 123
   behavioral/social research, 83
   biomedical research, basic, 53
   clinical research, 67
   homeostasis research, 49
   professional education, 40
   see also Centers of Excellence in Geriatric and Gerontological Research and Training
National Institute of Child Health and Human Development, 5, 34
National Institute of Mental Health, 5
National Institutes of Health, 5, 26, 28, 29–30, 103, 119–120, 121
   behavioral/social research, 20, 83
   biomedical research, basic, 52
   clinical research, 16
   ethical issues, 24
Neoplasia, see Cancer; Tumors, benign
Neurosciences, 5, 50
   aging, general, 10, 66

INDEX

behavioral, 18, 73, 76
brain, 10, 18, 73, 84–85
cellular, 11, 50
endocrinology, 11, 50, 76
pain, 16, 66
postural/mobility disorders, 13, 60–61
sensory deficiencies, 13, 16, 77
urinary incontinence, 14, 62
see also Dementia
Nonprofit organizations, *see* Foundations
Nursing homes, 7, 93–94, 124, 126
costs, 8
ethical issues, 109, 110, 114–115
mental disorders, 99
urinary incontinence, 14
Nutrition, 16, 51
genetics and, 63, 66
musculoskeletal disorders, 15

O

Oral cavity, *see* Dental and oral diseases
Osteoarthritis, 10, 15, 49, 54, 64
Osteoporosis, 8, 15, 59, 64, 127
Our Future Selves, 43

P

Pain, 16, 66
Panel for Statistics for an Aging Population, 91
Pepper Commission, 26
see also Centers of Excellence in Geriatric and Gerontological Research and Training
Pew Charitable Trusts, vii, 123
Pharmacological agents, 3, 21, 89
costs, 96, 98
epidemiology, 103
ethical issues, 69
medication mismanagement, 13–14, 21, 51, 61, 96–97, 101
polypharmacy, 61, 97
private sector, 143
standards, 63
Pneumonia, 65
Postural stability, 13, 60–61
Poverty, 2, 18, 74, 78, 93, 95, 113
Preventive medicine, *see* Health promotion
Private sector, 26, 122, 143
innovation, 36–37
see also Foundations

Professional education, 4–5, 6, 31–32, 36, 40, 41, 124, 127–130
academic research, 4–5, 124, 129–130
behavioral/social, 20
biomedical, 12, 24, 54
clinical, 16, 67–68
health services, 88–89, 93, 103
multidisciplinary approach, 24, 55
Prostate gland, 10, 49, 54
Psychology and psychiatry, 16, 45, 46, 63–64, 76, 78, 81, 85, 99–100
differential aging, 73–74, 77
disease, concomitants, 20, 103
research, priority, 17–18
research, secondary, 20
see also Mental health and illness
Publications, 40–41, 43, 125–127, 128, 129
see also specific publications

Q

Quality of life, 2, 4, 6, 7–8, 9, 89
drug mismanagement and, 61
index of, 19–20, 80–81
long-term care, 91, 92, 94
quality of care *vs*, 24, 92, 94, 115
social factors, 19
see also Dependence/independence

R

Race/ethnicity, 17, 25, 45, 53, 68, 72, 74, 78, 79, 84, 95, 103
Regulations
drugs, 21
see also Standards
Rehabilitation, 13, 57, 58–59, 76, 111
Reproductive system, 51
Retirement, 19, 76–77, 79–80, 82
Risk factors, 13, 22, 55, 59, 96, 100, 102
cognitive impairments, 18
dementia, 99
social, 18, 79
Robotics, 22

S

Self-care, *see* Dependence/independence
Sensory deficiencies, 13, 16, 77
Sex differences, *see* Gender differences; Women
Skin diseases, 16, 66

Social sciences and services, 2, 3, 16, 25, 45, 46, 71–75, 127, 138–139
  cultural factors, 17, 25, 45, 53, 72–73, 77–78, 84
  differential aging, 17, 51, 71, 72, 73–74, 77
  drug effects, 21
  funding, 20, 30, 82–83
  longitudinal studies, 17, 19, 71, 81, 82, 83
  long-term care, 95
  methodology, 81–82
  multidisciplinary approach, 25, 46, 58, 71, 72, 73, 81–82, 83–85
  research, priority, 18–19, 75–80
  research, secondary, 19–20, 80–81
  risk factors, general, 18, 79
  technological innovations, effects, 19, 80, 94
  see also Demographic factors; Employment and unemployment; Families
Socioeconomic status, 78, 79, 84, 103
  and allocation of health care resources, 95
  poverty, 2, 18, 74, 78, 93, 95, 113
Standards
  of care, 24, 111
  drugs, 63
  equity and access, 111–112
  long-term care, 94
  see also Biomedical ethics

T

Technological innovation
  behavioral/social effects, 19, 80, 94
  ethical issues, 24
  effectiveness, 22, 94
  imaging, 15
  industry support, 36–37
  long-term care, 94
Tissue studies, 11, 53, 55
Toward an Independent Old Age: A National Plan for Research on Aging, 2, 3, 43
Tumors, benign, 54
  prostatic, 10, 49, 54

U

Urinary system
  incontinence, 14, 61–62
  infections, 65

V

Vaccines, 15, 65

W

Weingart Foundation, 123
Women, 74, 79, 95
  hypertension, 25, 68
  osteoporosis, 8
  workforce, 89, 93
  see also Gender differences

WITHDRAWN

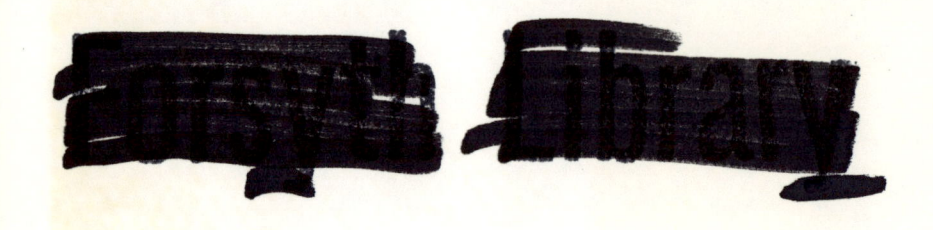